Exercises in Pregnancy and Childbirth

A Practical Guide for Educators

LI

T

For Books for Midwives:

Senior Commissioning Editor: Mary Seager
Development Editor: Catharine Steers
Project Manager: Joannah Duncan
Designer: George Ajayi
Illustration Manager: Bruce Hogarth

Exercises in Pregnancy and Childbirth
A Practical Guide for Educators

Eileen Brayshaw MSc MCSP, SRP, FETC
Clinical Associate, Huddersfield University,
Clinical Specialist and Postgraduate Physiotherapy Tutor
in Women's Health

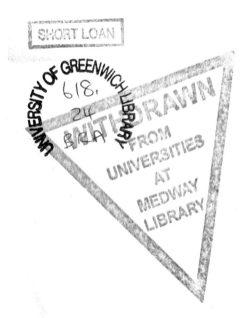
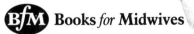 **Books *for* Midwives**

EDINBURGH LONDON NEW YORK OXFORD PHILADELPHIA ST LOUIS SYDNEY TORONTO 2003

BOOKS FOR MIDWIVES
An imprint of Elsevier Science Limited

First published 2003

ISBN 0 7506 5600 X

British Library Cataloguing in Publication Data
A catalogue record for this book is available from the British Library

Library of Congress Cataloging in Publication Data
A catalog record for this book is available from the Library of
Congress

Notice
Medical knowledge is constantly changing. Standard safety
precautions must be followed, but as new research and clinical
experience broaden our knowledge, changes in treatment and
drug therapy may become necessary or appropriate. Readers are
advised to check the most current product information provided by
the manufacturer of each drug to be administered to verify the
recommended dose, the method and duration of administration, and
contraindications. It is the responsibility of the practitioner, relying on
experience and knowledge of the patient, to determine dosages and
the best treatment for each individual patient. Neither the Publisher
nor the author assumes any liability for any injury and/or damage to
persons or property arising from this publication.

The Publisher

**ELSEVIER
SCIENCE**
your source for books,
journals and multimedia
in the health sciences
www.elsevierhealth.com

The
publisher's
policy is to use
**paper manufactured
from sustainable forests**

Printed in China

Contents

Preface **vii**

History of physical preparation for childbirth **ix**

1. Pelvic anatomy **1**

2. Physiological changes and common physical problems in pregnancy **15**

3. Musculoskeletal problems in pregnancy and postpartum **25**

4. Antenatal exercises and advice **41**

5. Stress and relaxation **57**

6. Coping strategies for labour **69**

7. Transcutaneous electrical nerve stimulation (TENS) **83**

8. Physiological changes and physical problems in the puerperium **91**

9. Postnatal exercises and advice **101**

10. Teaching exercises **117**

11. Programme planning for physical skills **143**

12. Alternative approaches to fitness antenatally and postpartum **153**

Appendix: Suppliers of equipment and information **171**

Index **175**

Preface

This comprehensive guide to exercise and relaxation for pregnancy, birth and postpartum replaces *Teaching Physical Skills for the Childbearing Year*, written by Eileen Brayshaw and Pauline Wright in 1994. This earlier book was produced in response to requests from midwives, health visitors and others involved in the teaching of physical preparation for childbirth without the help of a women's health physiotherapist. It was also of value to students and rotational physiotherapists who had no specific experience in obstetrics.

Since the publication of *Teaching Physical Skills for the Childbearing Year*, much research has been published about appropriate abdominal exercises during pregnancy and postpartum. Some of the exercises, which were considered standard in the early nineties, have now been revised and Chapters 4, 9 and 10 of this book reflect this new approach to evidence-based exercises for the childbearing year. Also included is a separate chapter on the musculoskeletal problems which present during pregnancy and/or postpartum (Ch. 3). This is an area that is not covered in detail by midwives or health visitors during their training. Information on characteristic symptoms and advice about when to refer on to a women's health physiotherapist is offered.

Many childbirth educators lack the expertise and background knowledge required to enable them to teach exercise and relaxation with confidence. They should understand the rationale for including these skills in the preparation for parenthood, before attempting to teach them. Incorporated in this guide is a basic description of the relevant physiology, and of the anatomy and functions of those joints and muscles especially involved during the childbearing year. Having gained this knowledge the reader can then move on to the subsequent chapters to learn and practise performing the basic exercises, relaxation and coping strategies for labour. Later chapters describe how to teach these physical skills to individuals and small groups and how they may be incorporated into different preparation programmes.

The exercises are intentionally repeated in both the ante- and postnatal sections so that each chapter can stand independently. Chapter 10 embraces all the information relating to the exercises in Chapters 4 and 9 in a comprehensive package for easy referral. The final chapter on alternative approaches to overall fitness has been extensively updated as this is an area where much advice is sought by women. It now includes an overview of Pilates for pregnancy and postpartum.

An accompanying CD Rom incorporates the content of Chapters 5 and 10.

Finally I would like to thank Georgina, Helen and Julie for their advice, and Sue and Jo for their unfailing help and support.

Eileen Brayshaw
Leeds, 2003

History of physical preparation for childbirth

As far back as 1912 Minnie Randell, head of St. Thomas's School of Physiotherapy, and also a midwife, was asked by Dr. Fairbairn, an obstetrician, to teach postnatal exercises in order to aid physical recovery and encourage rest and relaxation. A physical routine was then established antenatally to promote physical health and help prevent problems. Minnie Randell was further influenced by Dr. Kathleen Vaughan, who encouraged the teaching of stretching exercises to increase the mobility of the pelvic joints and lumbar spine. Positions of comfort were also introduced to facilitate labour.

From the 1930s, the pioneer, Grantly Dick-Read, voiced his theory of the fear-tension-pain cycle in labour. He included very little general exercise in his training programme, but emphasis was placed on women learning to relax and breathe deeply through contractions. Minnie Randell followed this regime and in partnership with Margaret Morris, a ballet dancer, encouraged women to rehearse for the performance of labour. Helen Heardman, another teacher of physiotherapy, based her teaching on ideas from both St. Thomas's and Grantly Dick-Read. In the 1940s she offered courses on labour and parenthood, which included education, relaxation and breathing.

In the 1950s, psychoprophylaxis became fashionable. This was a new trend, which came to Britain from Russia via Paris. A very rigid training was taught and included controlled patterns (levels) of breathing. It was only a preparation for labour; postnatal rehabilitation was not included as part of the course.

In common with other forms of education, there has been a move from authoritarian didactic teaching to a client-led approach. Both women and partners now attend psychophysical preparation classes and express their physical and emotional needs for inclusion in the programme. Relaxation, breathing and exercises are always requested. This book concentrates on these.

Over the years there have been discussions between the Royal College of Midwives, the Health Visitors Association and the Chartered Society of Physiotherapy about each member's role in Psychophysical Preparation, and the latest tripartite agreement (1994) is as follows: *working together in psychophysical preparation for childbirth.*

1. Midwives, health visitors and [1]obstetric physiotherapists all have important specialist contributions to make in the preparation for childbirth and parenthood. This contact with parents also provides a valuable opportunity for more general health promotion, health education and preventative medicine. In the delivery of such a service in any locality, it is important that the professional team demonstrates a flexible approach and takes account of the views and needs of all parents.

2. The role of the midwife is that of the practitioner of normal midwifery, caring for the woman within the hospital and community throughout the continuum of pregnancy, childbirth and the puerperium. She has an important contribution to make in health education, counselling and support. In this context her aim is to facilitate the realisation of women's needs, discuss expectations and air anxieties. She has the responsibility of monitoring the woman's physical, psychological and social wellbeing and is in a unique position to be able to correlate parent education with midwifery care.

3. The role of the health visitor in this field is to offer advice to the parents-to-be on the many health, psychological and social implications of becoming parents, and the development of the child. She is in a very special position in the family scene to inform them of the services available and to encourage them to use them. The health visitor should always have a participatory role within the team to provide continuity of care to the family.

4. The role of the women's health physiotherapist is to promote health during the childbearing period and to help the woman adjust advantageously to the physical and psychological changes of pregnancy and the postnatal period so that the stresses of childbearing are minimised. Antenatally and postnatally she advises on physical activity associated with both work and leisure, and is a specialist in selecting and teaching appropriate exercises to gain and/or maintain fitness including pelvic floor education. Where necessary she gives specialised treatment, e.g. therapeutic ultrasound, postnatally to alleviate discomfort. She also assesses and treats musculoskeletal problems such as backache and pelvic floor muscle weakness. In addition she is a skilled teacher of effective relaxation, breathing awareness and positioning, and thus helps the woman to prepare for labour.

---

[1]In 1997 The Association of Chartered Physiotherapists in Obstetrics and Gynaecology (ACPOG) changed its name to the Association of Chartered Physiotherapists in Women's Health (ACPWH). Where an obstetric physiotherapist is stated it should be replaced by the term women's health physiotherapist.

5. In order for the services of the team to be of maximum benefit to parents there should be a close liaison between its members. Liaison, planning and shared learning sessions help to ensure that techniques and advice are consistent and up-to-date, relate to current practice and meet the needs of the parents. This is particularly important when there is no available member of one of the specialist professions. Where this is the case, advice should be sought from the relevant professional body. To enhance continuity of care, new members of the team must always have a period of inter-disciplinary induction. The midwife, health visitor and obstetric physiotherapist should be in regular contact and operate an effective referral system.
6. The aims of parenthood education are summarised as follows:
   - to enable parents to develop a confident and relaxed approach to pregnancy, childbirth and parenthood
   - to enable parents to be aware of the choices in care based on accurate and up-to-date information
   - to provide continuity of high quality care, as previously defined to parents, by means of team collaboration and cooperation between professionals, including specialised treatments where needed
   - to ensure that appropriate, consistent and clear advice is given with full cognisance of safety factors
   - to promote health and preventative medicine.

Frequently new methods of education in parenthood are introduced, e.g. aquanatal and fitness classes. In such instances it is necessary for guidance to be sought from the local obstetric physiotherapist or alternatively from the Chartered Society of Physiotherapy, and further training may be required.

1

Pelvic anatomy

The pelvis 01
  Stability of the spine and pelvis 02
  Anatomical relations 03
The abdominal wall 04
  Linea alba 04
  Transversus abdominis 04
  Internal oblique 05
  External oblique 07
  Rectus abdominis 08
  The rectus sheath 08
  Pyrimidalis 09
  Multifidus 09

Thoracolumbar fascia 10
Nerve supply 11
Combined functions of the
  abdominal muscles 11
The pelvic floor 11
  Superficial perineal muscles 11
  Levator ani 12
  Pelvic floor fascia 13
  Nerve supply 13
  Combined functions of the pelvic
    floor muscles 13
References 14

This chapter contains the relevant anatomy for background knowledge when teaching physical skills in preparation for parenthood.

THE PELVIS

The pelvis is the bony ring at the base of the trunk. It is made up of four bones – the coccyx, sacrum and two large innominate or hip bones (Figure 1.1). Three parts make up each innominate bone – the ilium, ischium and pubis. The sacrum, a wedge-shaped bone made up of five rudimentary sacral vertebrae, joins the two iliac bones at the part-synovial, part-fibrous sacroiliac joints. The joint joining the two pubic bones anteriorly is the cartilaginous symphysis pubis and the coccyx (usually composed of four rudimentary coccygeal vertebrae) is attached to the sacrum at the sacrococcygeal joint. As well as these joints linking the bones of the pelvis together, the rest of the spine is attached to the sacrum at the lumbar sacral joint. Ligaments, strong bands of fibrous tissue consisting of fibroblasts and tightly packed bundles of collagen fibres, surround the joints and are normally limited in their flexibility in order to protect the joints and restrict unwanted movement (Figure 1.2).

The pelvis protects the abdominal viscera, provides muscle attachments and transmits weight to the lower limbs in standing and walking.

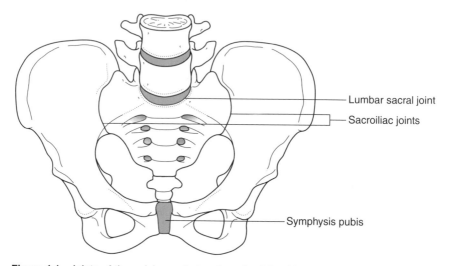

Figure 1.1 Joints of the pelvis – anterior view of pelvis with lumbar vertebrae.

Stability of the spine and pelvis

Panjabi (1992) states that spinal stability relies on the coordinated interaction of three subsystems:

1. the control subsystem which includes all neural structures
2. the passive subsystem which includes the vertebrae, intervertebral discs, ligaments, joint capsules and fascia
3. the active subsystem which includes all the muscles and their tendons.

   As these subsystems rely on each other, any dysfunction in any one subsystem will affect the overall stability of the spine.

   Vleeming et al (1995) believe that stability of the pelvis relies on a self-locking mechanism which is the inter-relationship of the form and force closing mechanisms of the pelvis. The form closure relates to the articular surfaces held together by ligaments, whilst the force closure is that created by the effectiveness and balance of the surrounding abdominal and back muscles. Hormonal influences in pregnancy affect the pliability of the ligamentous tissue leading to slightly increased movements in the joints of the pelvis (see Ch. 2). This increases the transverse and antero-posterior diameters of the pelvic outlet, which will be of advantage during labour and delivery (see Ch. 6). However, increased joint mobility may also contribute to spinal and pelvic instability and cause pain not only during pregnancy but long-term (Watkins 1998).

(a) Anterior view

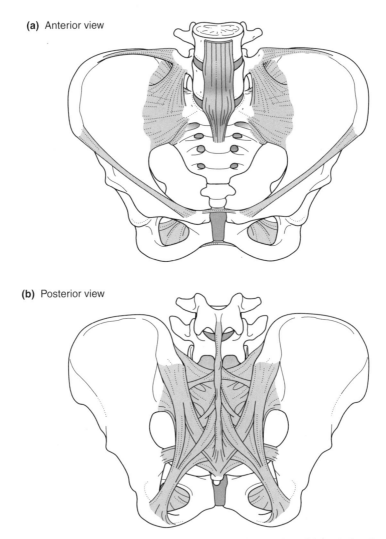

(b) Posterior view

Figure 1.2 The pelvis showing the ligaments: (a) anterior view; (b) posterior view.

Anatomical relations

The abdominal cavity extends from the diaphragm down to the pelvic floor. It can be described as a capsule formed by the abdominal muscles anteriorly, back muscles posteriorly, diaphragm superiorly and the pelvic floor muscles inferiorly (Hodges 1999). Within the pelvic area of the cavity, the uterus and the vagina lie between the bladder and the urethra in front, and the rectum and anus behind. The uterus projects into the vagina almost horizontally when a woman is in the standing position. It is held in position by ligaments and, indirectly, by the pelvic floor. It is movable, for example, when a full bladder pushes it into a vertical position. During pregnancy the uterus enlarges and its position changes. It rises out of the pelvis and the upper part reaches the sternum by about 36 weeks gestation. During the last month of pregnancy the level falls when the fetal head descends into the pelvis. The growing uterus puts pressure on the bladder and bowel, which can lead to increased urinary frequency and intestinal discomfort.

THE ABDOMINAL WALL

The abdominal wall can be likened to a human corset and it comprises four sets of abdominal muscles and fascia on each side of the body. Three of these are flat muscles arranged in layers covering the anterior and lateral areas of the trunk. The fibres of each muscle end in an aponeurosis – a flat, thin tendon which spreads out in the form of a broad sheet; most of the anterior abdominal wall is aponeurotic rather than muscular. The flat abdominal muscles are the transversus abdominis and the internal and external obliques. The fourth set, the rectus abdominis, is a band-like muscle lying on either side of the linea alba anteriorly.

Linea alba

The linea alba is a fascial thickening with criss-cross fibres in the midline, extending from the xiphoid process down to the pubic symphysis. It is 1–2 cms wide above the umbilicus and only 1 cm below the umbilicus. Like the pelvic ligaments, it is under the influence of the relaxing hormones during pregnancy and will stretch both widthways and lengthways (see Ch. 2).

Transversus abdominis

The deepest muscle of the abdominal corset is the transversus abdominis (transversus) which arises from the thoracolumbar fascia, the iliac crest and the inguinal ligament and above from the inner surfaces of the costal cartilages of the six lower ribs, interdigitating with the origin of the diaphragm. The muscle fibres run mainly horizontally forwards and end in an aponeurosis which takes part in the formation of the rectus sheath, (described later) and then attaches itself to the length of the linea alba (see Figure 1.3). The lower fibres arising from the inguinal ligament curve downwards to join with the inferior fibres of the internal oblique muscle to form the conjoint tendon.

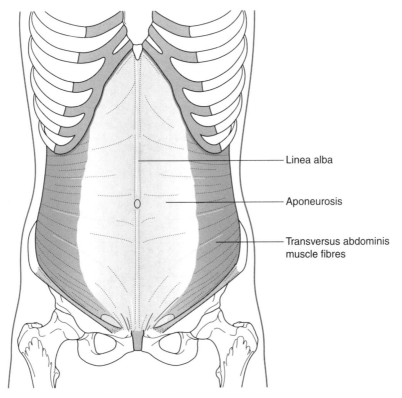

Figure 1.3 Transversus abdominis.

Actions

Because of its deep situation and its origin within the thoracolumbar fascia, the transversus muscle is now recognized as being the prime stabilizer of the trunk (Hodges 1999) and works with multifidus. It helps to stabilize the linea alba during trunk flexion. The anterior fibres work with the lower anterior fibres of the internal oblique to compress and support the abdominal viscera. The upper fibres help to decrease the infrasternal angle of the ribs in expiration.

Internal oblique

The internal oblique is a broad thin sheet lying between the transversus and the external oblique. It arises from the thoracolumbar fascia, the iliac crest and the inguinal ligament. It runs mainly upwards and forwards and the highest posterior fibres are inserted into the cartilages of the lower

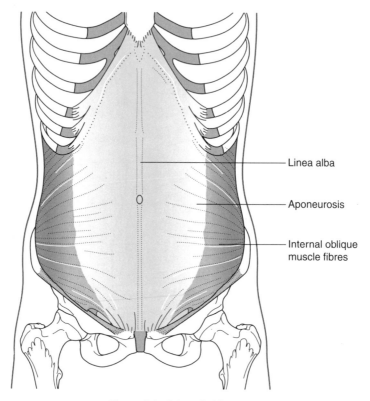

Figure 1.4   Internal oblique.

three ribs. The rest of the muscle fibres spread out and become an aponeurosis. This again takes part in the formation of the rectus sheath and is then attached to the xiphoid process, 7th, 8th and 9th costal cartilages, costal margin, linea alba and pubic crest (see Figure 1.4). The inferior fibres join with the lower fibres of the transversus to form the conjoint tendon.

Actions

Working bilaterally, the upper anterior fibres assist in flexion of the spine. Unilaterally they work with the anterior fibres of the external oblique muscle on the opposite side to rotate the spine. When the pelvis is fixed, the right internal oblique and the left external oblique muscles rotate the thorax to the right and vice versa. The lower anterior fibres work with transversus abdominis and compress and support the abdominal viscera. The lateral fibres work with the lateral fibres of the external oblique on the same side to flex the spine sideways.

External oblique

The external oblique is also a wide thin sheet of muscle with fibres generally running at right angles to those of the internal oblique. The fibres run obliquely downwards and inwards in the direction in which one would put one's hands into trouser pockets. The muscle fibres arise from the outer surfaces of the lower eight ribs by slips which interdigitate with the serratus anterior and latissimus dorsi muscles. This arrangement may be seen in well-developed subjects. The muscle fibres radiate downwards and forwards. The lowest posterior fibres pass vertically downwards and are inserted into the iliac crest. The rest of the fibres form an extensive triangular aponeurosis which is attached to the anterior superior iliac spine, the pubic tubercle and crest and the linea alba. The lower margin of the external oblique aponeurosis is folded back on itself between the anterior superior iliac spine and the pubic tubercle and forms the tendinous inguinal ligament. The anterior part of the aponeurosis helps to form the rectus sheath (see Figure 1.5).

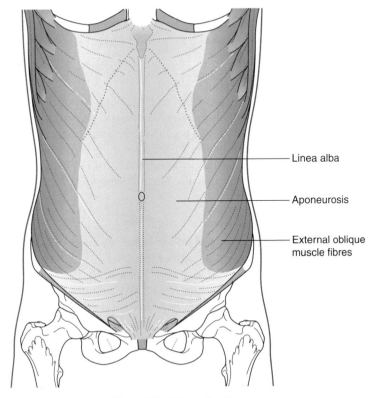

Figure 1.5 External oblique.

Actions

Working bilaterally, the anterior fibres work with rectus abdominis to tilt the pelvis posteriorly. The posterior fibres work with rectus abdominis to flex the spine. Unilaterally the muscle works with the internal oblique muscles to rotate and side flex the spine (see earlier text).

Rectus abdominis

The most anterior and superficial of the abdominal muscles is the rectus abdominis (rectus). The muscle is long and strap-like and is located on either side of the midline. It is attached to the outer, anterior part of the ribcage, the anterior aspect of the 5th, 6th and 7th costal cartilages and the xiphoid process. The muscle narrows as the fibres pass straight down the abdomen to divide into two tendons. The medial head is attached to the ligaments in front of the symphysis pubis, many of the fibres attaching themselves to the opposite side. The lateral head is attached to the pubic crest of its own side. On the anterior surface of the muscle, but not extending through the entire substance of the muscle, are three (or more) transverse tendinous intersections at and above the umbilicus, which are firmly adherent to the anterior wall of the muscle sheath. These may be seen as transverse grooves on well-developed muscular male subjects (see Figure 1.6).

Actions

Rectus abdominis, working with the internal and external obliques and psoas, flexes the spine approximating the thorax and pelvis. It also assists the obliques and back extensors in side flexion of the spine. Because of its pubic attachment, it lifts the front of the pelvis (working together with gluteus maximus), thus counteracting the forward tilting of the pelvis that causes lumbar lordosis. Rectus abdominis also supports the symphysis pubis.

The rectus sheath

The rectus abdominis is wrapped in an envelope of fascia derived from the aponeuroses of the other abdominal muscles – the rectus sheath. The external oblique passes in front of the rectus sheath, the internal oblique separates to enclose it, and the transversus abdominis passes behind. The sheath can stretch lengthways but less so crossways. Above the costal margin (see Figure 1.7a), only the anterior wall of the sheath is present; it is made up entirely by the external oblique aponeurosis. Posteriorly, the rectus lies on the ribs and intercostal muscles. In the lower part of the abdomen (see Figure 1.7b), all three aponeuroses lie over the front of the rectus, the posterior wall being formed only by the fascia which lines the inside of the abdominal wall.

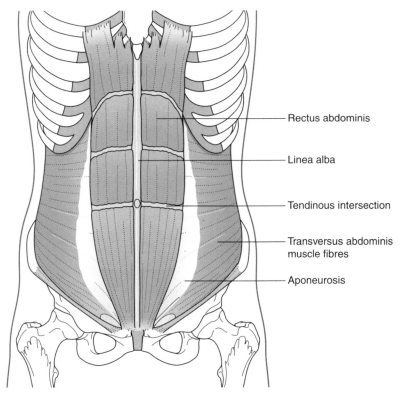

Figure 1.6 Rectus abdominis.

Pyrimidalis

A small triangular muscle, the pyramidalis, lies inside the rectus sheath, in front of the lower part of the rectus. It originates from the anterior surface of the pubis and attaches itself to the linea alba. Its action is to tighten the linea alba. Pyramidalis is not always present and its absence may be implicated in diastasis of the rectus abdominis muscles (see Ch. 3) seen below the umbilicus (Boissonnault & Kotarinos 1988).

Multifidus

Multifidus is the deepest of the back muscles beneath semispinalis and erector spinae, lying in the gutter between the spinous and transverse processes of the vertebrae at all levels of the spine. The lumbar section arises from the back of the sacrum and the fascia covering erector spinae and the mamilliary processes of the lumbar vertebrae. The fibres are in

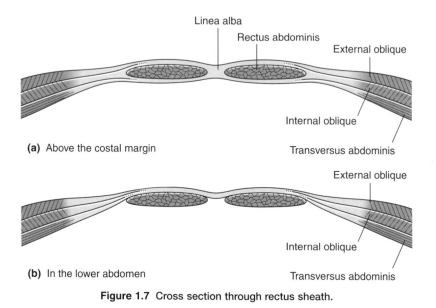

Figure 1.7 Cross section through rectus sheath.

three layers and attach to the spines of all the vertebrae. The deepest layer passes upwards and medially to the vertebra above, the middle layer passes to the next but one vertebra, whilst the outer layer passes up to the third or fourth vertebra above.

Actions

The lumbar section of multifidus is an important stabilizer of the pelvis working with transversus abdominis, and allows efficient action of the long muscles. It also produces rotation, extension and lateral flexion of the spine.

Thoracolumbar fascia

The thoracic component of the thoracolumbar fascia is a fairly thin layer attached to the spines of the vertebrae and the angles of the ribs. The lumbar component has three layers. The posterior layer is attached to the spines of the lumbar and sacral vertebrae and to the supraspinous ligament. The middle layer is attached to the transverse processes of the lumbar vertebrae, the intertransverse ligaments, the iliac crest, the lower borders of the 12th rib and the lumbocostal ligament. The anterior layer is attached to the transverse processes of the lumbar vertebrae, the iliolumbar ligament and iliac crest. The posterior and middle layers unite and join with the anterior layer laterally to form the origin of transversus abdominis.

Nerve supply

The lower six thoracic nerves supply the abdominal muscles. The oblique and transversus muscles are also supplied by the iliohypogastric and ilioinguinal nerves. Multifidus is supplied by the posterior rami of the spinal nerves.

Combined functions of the abdominal muscles:

- support the abdominal contents in position partly by mechanical action and partly by maintaining intra-abdominal pressure
- support and control the spine in posture, movement and load-bearing activities
- with the diaphragm and pelvic floor muscles – increase the intra-abdominal pressure and thus assist with all expulsive efforts such as coughing, micturition, defaecation, vomiting and parturition
- effect movements of the trunk – flexion, side flexion and rotation

Transversus and the obliques play the major part in spinal support and control providing a dynamic corset-like structure for fixation and support (Richardson & Jull 1995).

Weakness of the abdominal and back muscles may lead to instability of the pelvis and disruption of the load transfer from the pelvis to the lower limbs (see Ch. 3) and can lead to long-term pain (Watkins 1998).

THE PELVIC FLOOR

The pelvic floor forms a base to the pelvis and is composed of the superficial perineal muscles, fascia and the deeper levator ani and coccygeus muscles.

Superficial perineal muscles

Superficial perineal muscles consist of small thin bands of striated muscle radiating outwards to the pelvic bones at each side from the central tendinous perineal body. The perineal body is a pyramid of muscle and fibrous tissue and is situated between the vagina and the rectum. Bulbospongiosus is attached to the perineal body round the vagina to the clitoris. Ischiocavernosus is attached to the ischial tuberosity and clitoris. The superficial transverse perineal muscles attach the ischial tuberosities to the perineal body. The external anal sphincter surrounds the anal orifice and is embedded in front of the perineal body and attaches itself behind the coccyx (see Figure 1.8).

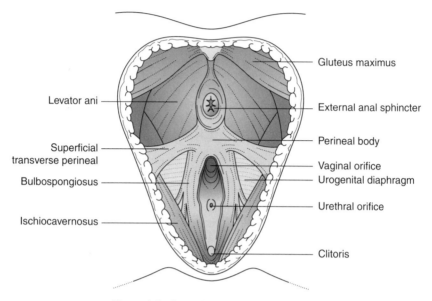

Figure 1.8 Superficial pelvic floor muscles.

Levator ani

This deep layer of muscles can be considered as one sheet of muscle covered by pelvic fascia; it forms a strong sling supporting the abdominal viscera. The muscles can be divided into ischiococcygeus (sometimes known as coccygeus), iliococcygeus, pubococcygeus and puborectalis and are attached to the pelvic surface of the pubic bone, obturator internus fascia and pelvic surface of the ischial spine. The muscle fibres pass with varying degrees of obliquity across the side of the vagina to be attached in the perineal body. Ischiococcygeus is a small triangular muscle, which is posterior and superior to, but in the same plane as, the rest of the levator ani, but it is sometimes considered as separate. It arises from the ischial spine and sacrospinous ligament and passes to the upper part of the coccyx and lower part of the sacrum. Iliococcygeus arises from the fascia over obturator internus and the ischial spine. The medial puborectalis fibres run either side of the urethra and vagina before being inserted into the perineal body, and the lateral fibres on each side encircle the rectum and blend with the external anal sphincter. It arises from the ischial spine and attaches itself onto the coccyx and lower sacrum (see Figure 1.9). Pubococcygeus arises from the pubic bone and fascia over obturator internus and attaches to the anterior surface of the coccyx.

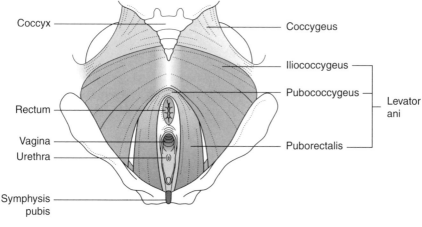

Figure 1.9 Deep pelvic floor muscles.

Pelvic floor fascia

A double sheet of fascia, the urogenital triangle or urogenital diaphragm, fills the triangular space below the symphysis pubis and the pubic rami. It is perforated in the middle to give passage to the vagina and urethra. The fascia also envelops the levator ani. It contains a few muscle fibres, namely the compressor urethrae and the deep transverse perineal. The latter is attached to the perineal body and helps to support and stabilise it. The fascia envelops and gives attachment to the muscles and is liable to be very stretched during childbirth.

Nerve supply

The above muscles are supplied by the pudendal plexus formed from the 2nd, 3rd, 4th and sometimes 5th sacral nerve routes (S2–5).

Combined functions of the pelvic floor muscles:

- forms a base to the outlet of the pelvis
- important in pelvic stability together with transversus abdominis
- supports the pelvic organs
- counteracts changes in abdominal pressure caused by such actions as coughing and lifting
- assists in maintaining continence

- allows micturition, defaecation and parturition
- produces a gutter to assist in the rotation of the fetal head during delivery
- plays a part in sexual enjoyment during intercourse.

The above functions are only performed efficiently if the muscles involved are maintained in a strong condition. Weakness of the pelvic floor muscles may contribute to urinary incontinence and prolapse of the uterus and/or vaginal walls (see Ch. 2).

REFERENCES

Boissonnault J J S, Kotarinos R K 1988 Diastasis recti. In: Wilder E (ed) Obstetric and Gynecologic Physical Therapy. Churchill Livingstone, Edinburgh
Hodges P W 1999 Is there a role for transversus abdominis in lumbo-pelvic stability? Manual Therapy 4(2):74–86
Panjabi M M 1992 The stability system of the spine. Part 1 Function, dysfunction, adaptation and enhancement. Journal of Spinal Disorders 5(4):383–396
Richardson C A, Jull G A 1995 Muscle control – pain control. What exercises would you prescribe? Manual Therapy 1(2):2–10
Vleeming A, Snijders C J, Stoeckart R et al 1995 A new light on low back pain. Proceedings of the 2nd Interdisciplinary World Congress on Low Back Pain 149–167
Watkins Y 1998 Current concepts in dynamic stabilization of the spine and pelvis: their relevance in obstetrics. Journal of the Association of Chartered Physiotherapists in Women's Health 83:16–26

2

Physiological changes and common physical problems in pregnancy

The respiratory system 15
The cardiovascular system 16
The musculoskeletal
  system 17
Some common physical
  problems in pregnancy 20
  Cramp 20
  Varicose veins 20

Symphysis pubis dysfunction
  (SPD) 20
Carpal tunnel syndrome 21
Rib-pain (stitch) 21
Stress incontinence 21
Tiredness (fatigue) 22
Low back pain 22
References 22

This chapter presents the extensive physical and physiological alterations that take place in a woman's body during pregnancy through the actions of oestrogen, progesterone and relaxin. These create challenges, which should never be minimized, and it is important to understand the effects on the woman's systems before teaching exercise.

THE RESPIRATORY SYSTEM

The changes to the respiratory system during pregnancy are both physiological and mechanical. The demand for oxygen is increased because the basal metabolic rate is raised, as is the mass of the woman. At term the amount of oxygen required is about 20% above normal. There is a similar increase in the amount of carbon dioxide exhaled. The higher level of progesterone increases the sensitivity of the respiratory centre in the medulla to carbon dioxide levels in the blood (Dale & Mullinax 1988). This brings about a slight increase in the respiratory rate and there is a reduction of about 25% in the maternal blood carbon dioxide tension. Since the respiratory centre responds not to a scarcity of oxygen but to a surfeit of carbon dioxide, it is this lowering of the level of carbon dioxide which causes pregnant women to become breathless on activity. They often complain of difficulty in breathing (dyspnoea) even early in their pregnancies (Patterson & Lindsay 1988). There is a gradual increase in tidal volume by up to 40%. However, since the vital capacity remains more or less unchanged, there is an increase in ventilation of the alveoli due to a reduction in the volume of residual air.

Pregnant women may also hyperventilate (Bush 1992). This often happens during labour due to voluntary or involuntary overbreathing. Carbon dioxide is exhaled too forcefully leading to lightheadedness, tingling in the lips, hands and feet, sweating, panic and anxiety. Later symptoms could include unconsciousness. Theoretically, maternal hyperventilation could affect an already compromised fetus. The symptoms can be relieved and the condition reversed if the woman breathes with her cupped hands (or a paper bag) over her nose and mouth, thus re-inhaling her exhaled carbon dioxide. This will restore the blood gases to their normal level. The teacher should be aware of the risks of hyperventilation and unpleasant side effects, and teach ways of avoiding it. Practice of breathing awareness and adaptations for labour should be done with breaks interspersed to prevent this occurring (see Ch. 6).

In many pregnant women the ascending uterus progressively obstructs the descent of the diaphragm. It may even force the diaphragm upwards by 4 cm or more towards the end of pregnancy (Polden & Mantle 1990). This upward pressure may also push the rib cage out sideways and forwards, stretching the pliable tissues of the costal joint, which results in rib-flare that may give rise to pain and discomfort along the anterior margin of the lower ribs (see p21). Occasionally there is associated thoracic back pain. The antero-posterior and transverse diameters increase by about 10 cm (Revelli et al 1992). The flaring results in greater movements in the mid-costal and apical regions of the chest. For this reason women often experience dyspnoea (breathlessness) even during mild exertion towards the end of their pregnancy.

THE CARDIOVASCULAR SYSTEM

The changes that occur in the cardiovascular system are impressive because they take place during a short space of time and there is complete restoration to the normal state after delivery.

The woman's blood volume increases by at least 40%. The plasma volume rises to a higher level than the red cell mass, causing the haemoglobin level to fall to about 12 g/l (Polden & Mantle 1990). The resultant dilution anaemia may be one of the reasons why women feel tired from the early weeks of pregnancy.

The heart is pushed upwards by elevation of the diaphragm. It increases in size by about 12% (Chamberlain & Morgan 2002) due to stretching of the heart to accommodate the extra blood, and to muscle hypertrophy. A study showed an increase in cardiac output from 4.9 to 7.2 litres/minute during pregnancy, the main rise being in the first trimester (Robson et al 1991). The rise in cardiac output is achieved mainly by increased heart rate with a small rise in stroke volume (Chamberlain & Morgan 2002).

The smooth muscle of the walls of the blood vessels is relaxed by progesterone. This causes a small rise in body temperature and, more importantly, improves the peripheral circulation of the pregnant woman. Despite the increase in blood volume brought about by this hypotonia, blood pressure does not normally alter significantly during pregnancy. However, due to the slight decrease that may occur during the second trimester, women may feel faint when standing for too long. Movement of the feet should be encouraged if standing. To avoid feeling dizzy, women should be reminded to take extra time when getting up from the lying position.

A pregnant woman may feel faint when lying on her back. This is due to the enlarging fetus compressing the aorta and inferior vena cava against the lumbar spine, and so restricting blood flow. This effect is known as pregnancy supine hypotensive syndrome and can be relieved by turning the woman onto her side and giving reassurance. Supine hypotension often occurs during the third trimester (Revelli et al 1992). However it has been suggested that it could occur anytime after the fourth month of pregnancy (Artal & Buckenmeyer 1995). Teachers should be aware of this syndrome and are advised to refrain from teaching exercise and relaxation in the supine position after the fourth month of pregnancy (ACOG 2002).

Varicosities and gravitational oedema may be brought about by various factors. These may include the increase of pressure within the abdomen caused by the enlarging uterus, the general increase of body weight, the slight reduction in vascular tone (brought about by progesterone) and changes in collagen structure (caused by progesterone and relaxin). Varicose veins of the legs and vulva, and haemorrhoids may appear in pregnancy or, if previously present, may be accentuated.

In late pregnancy there may be oedema in the ankles, feet and hands which may lead to joint stiffness and nerve compression syndromes, the most common of which is carpal tunnel syndrome (see p21).

THE MUSCULOSKELETAL SYSTEM

The hormonal influences which affect the musculoskeletal system are particularly important to recognize before teaching exercises both antenatally and postnatally.

It is suggested that oestrogen prepares sites for the action of relaxin. Relaxin is produced as early as two weeks into pregnancy and is at its highest level in the first trimester, but then falls by approximately 50% and remains at that level until delivery (Kristiansson et al 1996). Relaxin alters the composition of collagen, which is present in joint capsules, ligaments and fibrous connective tissue, for example, the linea alba, and intersections of the rectus abdominis muscle, the rectus sheath, thoracolumbar fascia and the fascia of the pelvic floor. The remodelled collagen has greater elasticity and extensibility; the joints are therefore laxer and the abdomen yields more. It has been suggested that, in a second pregnancy, the range of the joints is further increased but that in subsequent pregnancies no additional change is likely (Calguneri et al 1982). This laxity of the joints is gradually reduced after delivery, but the process may take up to six months before it is completed (Sharpe 1998). The main joints affected by relaxin, and so especially vulnerable, are those of the pelvis. The symphysis pubis may separate – diastasis symphysis pubis (see Ch. 3) and there can be increased movement in the sacroiliac joints. However, all joints are affected, the weight-bearing joints being especially susceptible to stress. Even the ligaments of the feet become lax and, with the additional weight of pregnancy, can cause discomfort. Pregnant women often complain of aching and flat feet. The costal inter-articular tissues become more pliable and permit the rib-flaring described earlier in this chapter.

As the uterus enlarges, the centre of gravity moves forwards and this causes the woman to alter her standing position. Her posture will depend on the strength of her muscles, her extra weight, laxity of her joints, tiredness and prepregnancy posture. There is often, but not always, exaggeration of the lumbar curve (lordosis) and compensatory curving of the thoracic spine (kyphosis). This can occur between the fourth and ninth months of pregnancy and persist until 12 weeks postnatally (Bullock-Saxton 1991). There may be rounding of the shoulders and protruding chin and the woman may lean back (see Figure 2.1).

The incorrect posture imposes extra strain and fatigue on the body, particularly the spine, pelvis and weight-bearing joints and may give rise to aches and pains. In a study, Bullock et al (1987) found that 88.2% of women experienced back pain at some stage of their pregnancies. When questioned between 14 and 22 weeks gestation, 62% of the women reported that they had already experienced back pain. This suggests that abdominal enlargement was not the cause, but that hormonal changes and their influences on soft tissues may be important factors in producing the pain. Low back pain is often experienced, the pain sometimes spreading into the buttocks, the thighs and down the legs (see Ch. 3). Sometimes there is also an increased tenderness or pain over the symphysis pubis which may sometimes become incapacitating (see symphysis pubis dysfunction in Ch. 3).

Additional pressure through the spinal column is caused by increased bodyweight, and stress to the joints results from increased torsion. The woman is often unbalanced and, the joints being more mobile, she is more prone to injury.

The abdominal wall has to adjust to accommodate the enlarging uterus and its muscle fibres stretch considerably. In a primigravida woman abdominal measurements can increase by up to 115% (Gilleard & Brown 1996). The linea alba, fibrous sheaths, aponeuroses and intersections are all composed of collagen and are made more supple by hormonal influence. The two muscle bellies of the rectus abdominis separate as pregnancy advances and the linea alba stretches widthways, but with a lordotic posture this separation may be more pronounced and known as diastasis recti (see Ch. 3).

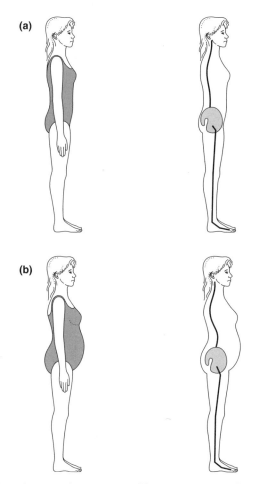

Figure 2.1   (a) Normal posture in pregnancy; (b) common posture in pregnancy showing increased lumbar lordosis.

The woman may experience a dragging, aching sensation in the lower abdomen as the weight of the uterus is transmitted through the abdominal muscles instead of those of the thighs and there may also be associated low-back pain. The strength of some muscles may actually increase during pregnancy as they have to support greater loads.

The enlarging uterus gradually increases pressure on the bladder, and the smooth muscle of the bladder and the urethra can lose tone due to the influence of progesterone (Chamberlain & Morgan 2002). It is also probable that the collagen present in the urethra and pelvic floor becomes more pliable. Hormonal action and increased weight during pregnancy can affect continence (see Ch. 3).

With all these widespread changes in the woman's body, it is evident that the healthier and fitter she is both before and during pregnancy, the more easily she will cope with pregnancy. Ideally, she should prepare physically for each pregnancy and maintain good health while she is pregnant. Recovery after delivery should then be quicker. Exercises and advice are included in preparation for parenthood sessions (see Ch. 4), but some women will request alternative approaches to fitness, for example, aerobic and aquanatal sessions or Pilates (see Ch. 12).

SOME COMMON PHYSICAL PROBLEMS IN PREGNANCY

Cramp

Cramp is very common during pregnancy and especially affects the calf muscles. Its cause is not known. Circulatory exercises (see Ch. 4) often help in preventing attacks and are to be encouraged, especially before sleep, as cramp often occurs at night. Stretching the leg and pointing the foot down (plantar flexion) often causes cramp so women must always remember to stretch with their feet pulled up (dorsiflexed). To alleviate cramp, the muscle should be put on a stretch by dorsiflexing the foot until the pain subsides.

Varicose veins

The varicose veins experienced by some women in pregnancy are caused by hormonal influence on the smooth muscle of the walls of the veins and the increased pressure within the abdomen. Circulatory exercises should improve venous return. In severe cases, support tights may be recommended. To be effective these must be put on even before the woman swings her legs over the side of the bed, otherwise the veins will already be distended. Prolonged standing and sitting with feet down or legs crossed can aggravate the condition.

Symphysis pubis dysfunction (SPD) (see Ch. 3)

This condition used to be referred to as diastasis symphysis pubis. Women with SPD will have pain and tenderness over the pubic area and down the inner thighs, which will vary in severity. Where possible the woman should be referred to a women's health physiotherapist. If the condition is acute, bed rest with the legs held closely together (adducted) and slightly bent over a thin pillow or folded towel, is essential. The woman may require a supporting belt (ideally a trochanteric belt – see appendix) or girdle and, when the pain is less severe, she could wear this for doing light housework. She can be advised to keep her legs together when she rolls over and to take small shuffling steps when she walks to reduce the discomfort. She may need a walking frame or crutches for support. The medical notes must have clear instructions about this condition as special management in labour (Fry 1999) will be required (see Ch. 6). Postnatal follow-up care by a women's health physiotherapist is essential.

Carpal tunnel syndrome

Carpal tunnel syndrome is the most common nerve-compression syndrome. It is caused by compression of the median nerve as it passes though the carpal tunnel at the wrist. It usually occurs after about 24 weeks if there is marked fluid-retention. Padua et al (2001) suggested that up to 62% of pregnant women have symptoms of this syndrome. Although it may be caused by localised oedema, it tends to be linked with generalised oedema. The woman often complains of numbness and stiffness in the fingers and she may find it difficult to pick up and hold small objects and to carry out small movements. This problem may be worse in the morning or at night when it may wake her. Wrist-splints can often give relief at night and can be worn during the day as well if needed (Courts 1995). In one survey, 46 out of 56 women became symptom-free by wearing wrist-splints at night (Ekman-Ordeberg et al 1987). The hands and arms should be supported in elevation when the woman is resting and she should be encouraged to perform wrist and hand exercises. Doing these in ice-cold water can sometimes give temporary relief. Women suffering from this condition should be warned to take extra care when handling hot liquids in a kettle, teapot or cup, especially first thing in the morning because they are more prone to accidents. Turgut et al (2001) found that the majority of women experienced spontaneous relief from their symptoms in the immediate postpartum period.

Rib-pain (stitch)

Women often experience a stitch-like pain along the lower anterior and lateral ribs. It may be caused by rib-flaring or by the stretching of the abdominal muscles. The problem can often be relieved by clasping the hands and stretching the arms above the head. Side-bending slightly away from the pain with the arm and hand above the head may also help but care should be taken to avoid leaning very far to one side. Some women find reverse sitting astride a chair comfortable (see Figure 6.1).

Stress incontinence (see Ch. 3)

It is suggested that in later pregnancy stress incontinence occurs in 50% of primigravidae and in nearly all multiparous women (Jolleys 1990). Marshall et al (1996) found that 40% of women reported some degree of leaking and that the incidence increased with parity. The problem should be discussed during antenatal classes and women reminded to perform regular pelvic floor exercises (see Ch. 4), it is never too late to start. Women with more severe stress incontinence should be referred to a women's health physiotherapist for individual assessment and treatment.

Tiredness (fatigue)

Women often feel very tired during the first trimester and again in the last three months as they become heavier. Ideally they will need to cut down their workloads, their partners being reminded to help out more with household tasks. This can be discussed in couples' sessions. Extra rest is essential and relaxation will be beneficial (see Ch. 5). Even if the woman is not complaining of tiredness, prevention is better than cure!

Low back pain (see Ch. 3)

In pregnancy the woman's weight has increased, she may be tired and may have poor posture. There will also be some instability of the joints caused by lax ligaments, altered spinal curves and stretched abdominal muscles. These and several other factors can lead to low-back pain. If acute, the first aid would be bed rest in a comfortable position, possibly side-lying with the top leg resting on a pillow between the legs (see Figure 5.3). At home, the woman may find comfort by placing a hot water bottle wrapped in towels against her back. Where possible she should be referred to a women's health physiotherapist for assessment and treatment.

When the pain is less severe, the woman can be shown gentle pelvic rocking (tilting). Advice should be given on such topics as positioning for rest, standing, walking and sitting posture, lifting, and advice on daily activities (see Ch. 4). The woman may find the back support of a pelvic girdle helpful (Bullock-Saxton 1998). The theme of back care should be continued postnatally (see Ch. 9).

REFERENCES

ACOG 2002 Committee Opinion: Exercise during pregnancy and the postpartum period. Obstetrics and Gynaecology 99(1):171–173
Artal R, Buckenmeyer P J 1995 Exercise during pregnancy and postpartum. Contemporary Obstetrics/Gynaecology 40(5):62–90
Bullock J E, Jull G A, Bullock M I 1987 The relationship of low back pain to postural changes during pregnancy. Australian Journal of Physiotherapy 33:10–17
Bullock-Saxton J E 1991 Changes in posture associated with pregnancy and the early postnatal period measured in standing. Physiotherapy Theory and Practice 7:103–109
Bullock-Saxton J 1998 Musculoskeletal changes in the perinatal period. In: Sapsford R, Bullock-Saxton J, Markwell S (eds) Women's Health. W B Saunders, London

Bush A 1992 Cardiopulmonary effects of pregnancy and labour. Journal of the Association of Chartered Physiotherapists in Obstetrics and Gynaecology 71:3–4

Calguneri M, Bird H A, Wright V 1982 Changes in joint laxity occurring during pregnancy. Annals of Rheumatic Diseases 41:126–128

Chamberlain G, Morgan M 2002 ABC of Antenatal Care, BMJ Books

Courts R B 1995 Splinting for symptoms of carpal tunnel syndrome during pregnancy. Journal of Hand Therapy 8(1):31–34

Dale F, Mullinax K M 1988 Physiologic adaptations and considerations of exercise during pregnancy. In: Wilder E (ed) Obstetric and Gynecologic Physical Therapy. Churchill Livingstone, Edinburgh

Ekman-Ordeberg G, Salgeback S, Ordeberg G 1987 Carpal tunnel syndrome in pregnancy. Acta Obstetrica et Gynaecolica Scandinavica 66:233–235

Fry D 1999 Perinatal symphysis pubis dysfunction: a review of the literature. Journal of the Association of Chartered Physiotherapists in Women's Health 85:11–18

Gilleard W L, Brown J M M 1996 Structure and function of the abdominal muscles in primigravid subjects during pregnancy and the immediate postbirth period. Physical Therapy 76(7):750–762

Jolleys J V 1990 The reported prevalence of urinary symptoms in women in one rural general practice. British Journal of General Practice 40(337):335–337

Kristiansson P, Svardsudd K, von Schoultz B 1996 Serum relaxin, symphyseal pain, and back pain during pregnancy. American Journal of Obstetrics and Gynecology 175(5):1342–1347

Marshall K, Totterdal D, McConnell V et al 1996 Urinary incontinence and constipation during pregnancy and after childbirth. Physiotherapy 82(2):98–103

Padua L, Aprile I, Caliandro P et al 2001 Symptoms and neurophysiological picture of carpal tunnel syndrome in pregnancy. Clinical Neurophysiology 112(10):1946–1951

Patterson C A, Lindsay M K 1988 Maternal Physiology in Pregnancy. In: Wilder E (ed). Obstetric and Gynecological Physical Therapy. Churchill Livingstone, Edinburgh

Polden M, Mantle J 1990 Physiotherapy in Obstetrics and Gynaecology. Butterworth-Heinemann, Oxford

Revelli A, Durando A, Massobrio M 1992 Exercise and Pregnancy: A Review of Maternal and Fetal Effects. Obstetrical and Gynecological Survey 47(6):355–367

Robson S C, Hunter S, Boys R et al 1991. Serial changes in haemodynamics during human pregnancy: a non-invasive study using Doppler echocardiography. Clinical Science 80:113–117

Sharpe R 1998 Pregnancy and the puerperium: Physiological changes. In: Sapsford R, Bullock-Saxton J, Markwell S (eds) Women's Health. Saunders, London

Turgut F, Cetinsahinahin M, Turgut M et al 2001 The management of carpal tunnel syndrome in pregnancy. Journal of Clinical Neuroscience 8(4):332–334

3

Musculoskeletal problems in pregnancy and postpartum

Low back pain (LBP) 25
  Treatment 26
Posterior pelvic pain (PPP) 27
  Treatment 28
Symphysis pubis dysfunction
  (SPD) 28
  Treatment during
    pregnancy 30
  During labour/delivery 30
  After delivery 30

Diastasis recti 31
  Rectus check 33
  Treatment 33
Pregnancy-associated osteoporosis
  (PAO) 34
Pelvic floor dysfunction 35
  Urinary incontinence 35
  Faecal incontinence 37
  Prolapse 37
References 38

This chapter highlights the presenting symptoms and basic treatment of the musculoskeletal problems which may manifest in pregnancy and which could lead to long-term problems if not recognised and referred to the appropriate professional. Some problems may even be avoided with the correct advice.

Musculoskeletal problems in pregnancy and postpartum include:

- low back pain (LBP)
- posterior pelvic pain (PPP)
- symphysis pubis dysfunction (SPD)
- diastasis recti
- pregnancy-associated osteoporosis (PAO)
- pelvic floor dysfunction.

LOW BACK PAIN (LBP)

Low back pain (LBP) is common in pregnancy with reported incidences varying from approximately 50% in the UK and Scandinavia (Mantle 1994, Östgaard et al 1991) to nearly 70% in Australia (Bullock-Saxton 1988). Mantle reported that 16% of women studied complained of severe back pain and 36% of the women in Östgaard et al's 1991 study reported significant back pain.

Predisposing factors include weight gain, rapid postural changes, previous back pain, repetitive strain/lifting, multiparity, high levels of relaxin (Östgaard et al 1991, Östgaard & Andersson 1991, Rungee 1993). Initial high levels of relaxin may explain why some women have backache and pelvic joint pain very early on in pregnancy before there is weight gain or any postural changes. Relaxin levels are at their highest in the first trimester (Kristiansson et al 1996). McEvoy et al (2001) found that previous back pain in pregnancy was a predictor of back pain in a subsequent pregnancy.

Postnatally, low back pain that has been a problem during pregnancy, usually subsides gradually, but it may persist after birth in some cases. Östgaard & Anderson (1992) reported that 7% of the women they studied suffered from severe back pain even 18 months after the birth. This persistent pain is very likely to be due to the combination of pelvic instability caused by lax ligaments, and muscle imbalance caused by stretching of the abdominal muscles and possible shortening of the back muscles.

MacArthur et al (1990) proposed a relationship between long-term backache postpartum and epidural anaesthesia in labour but Russell et al (1993) refuted this, claiming that the postpartum backache was postural. This postural backache is common following an epidural, as women do not appreciate when they are in an uncomfortable position during labour because of loss of sensation and therefore do not adjust their position. Breen et al (1994) also found no association between epidural anaesthesia and back pain and suggested that the pain women suffered after an epidural was probably due to musculoskeletal causes. Butler & Fuller (1998) studied 300 women who had received epidural anaesthesia during labour and noted an incidence of back pain of 30% most of which subsided over 14 days. However there was some persistent back pain in 8.5%. They concluded that a previous history of back pain increased the likelihood of postpartum back pain following epidural anaesthesia.

Severe back pain postpartum may be associated with a large diastasis of the recti due to lack of support from the abdominal muscles anteriorly (see p31).

Treatment

During pregnancy women complaining of back pain should be referred to a women's health physiotherapist for individual assessment. Postural advice and appropriate exercises will be given and, if necessary, a support belt provided. Advice on back care, rest positions and daily activities is essential. Electrotherapeutic pain-relieving modalities are all contraindicated during pregnancy; however a warm, not hot, bath may be comforting. Young & Jewell (2000) suggested that a specially shaped pillow placed under the waist in side-lying appears to help to reduce back pain and encourage sleep – a feather pillow could be used if the woman has no allergies.

Postnatal postural backache may be relieved by the performance of pelvic rocking exercises in lying and sitting (see Ch. 9) and women may benefit from a warm water bottle or warm baths. Advice on positions for activities such as feeding and bathing baby should be given (see Ch. 9). If back pain persists then the woman should be referred for individual assessment by a woman's health physiotherapist who will advise on the appropriate rehabilitation of the postural muscles to restore pelvic stability.

Box 3.1 summarises the advice that can be given to women suffering from low back pain.

Box 3.1   Advice for women suffering from low back pain

- if pain is severe, ask for a referral to a women's health physiotherapist
- make sure posture is correct in all working and resting positions
- ensure work surfaces and work stations are the correct height to prevent stooping
- contract transversus and the pelvic floor muscles before changing positions or performing activities
- get out of bed by bending knees, rolling over on to side keeping knees together
- avoid exercises such as curl-ups or sit-ups
- avoid lifting if possible but if necessary, use correct lifting/handling techniques
- sleep with a pillow under the waist in side-lying to prevent spine sagging
- sit in a supportive chair with folded towel behind the lumbar spine and feet on floor
- avoid doing too much, have frequent rests
- do not wear high heels.

POSTERIOR PELVIC PAIN (PPP)

The term posterior pelvic pain includes pain and dysfuntion of the sacro-iliac joints. During pregnancy it is caused by changes in relaxin levels in early pregnancy (Rungee 1993). However Damen et al (2001) found that increased joint laxity was not associated with PPP but that there was a relationship between asymmetrical sacroiliac joint laxity and PPP. It may co-exist with low back pain and/or symphysis pubis dysfunction and is characterised by a sharp pain over the sacroiliac joint on weight-bearing and on turning over in bed (Östgaard 1995), and can be reproduced by sacroiliac compression during assessment by a women's health physio-therapist. Pain may be referred into the buttock, the posterior thigh or occasionally into the anterior thigh. It is sometimes described as sciatica, but this is not accurate as the pain does not follow the course of the sciatic nerve down to the foot but is associated with mechanical pressure on one or more pelvic ligaments by the enlarged uterus. True sciatica is only found in 1% of pregnant women (Östgaard et al 1991). Occasionally a sub-luxation of the sacroiliac joint may occur causing acute pain and inability to weight-bear on that side. A women's health physiotherapist may be able to manipulate the subluxed joint but if laxity is excessive, then the problem will probably recur. A supporting sacroiliac belt may help as will rest if this is possible.

Treatment

Assessment of the back to exclude any back problems, followed by assessment of the sacro-iliac joints must be performed by a women's health physiotherapist. It may be appropriate in severe cases (for example, subluxation) for the physiotherapist to mobilise/manipulate the affected joint and provide some support in the form of a sacroiliac belt to keep the pelvis as closed as possible. Advice on posture in all positions whilst resting and working is important and the woman must be advised to avoid activities and positions that may exacerbate the pain. In lying, she needs to avoid the three quarters-lying recovery position (see Figure 4.7c) where the top knee is bent up in front of the other, and instead lie with a pillow between the legs to maintain a gap between the knees and feet (see Figure 4.7b). She must be reminded to roll over in bed with her knees bent and kept together in line with her shoulders (see Figure 4.8). Transversus and pelvic floor contractions are important to help the stability of the pelvis and should also be performed before any change of position.

Box 3.2 summarises the advice that can be given to women suffering from posterior pelvic pain.

Box 3.2 Advice for women suffering from posterior pelvic pain

---

- if pain is severe, ask for a referral to a women's health physiotherapist
- sleep in side-lying with a pillow lengthways between the legs
- avoid using the coma position
- contract transversus and the pelvic floor muscles before changing positions or performing activities
- roll over in bed by keeping knees and shoulders in line to avoid twisting
- avoid stooping or bending during activities
- do not sit with legs crossed
- avoid any positions or activities which cause/increase pain
- wear a pelvic support to improve pelvic stability.

SYMPHYSIS PUBIS DYSFUNCTION (SPD)

SPD is a term used that encompasses altered function of the symphysis pubis joint and pain experienced around the area of the joint. It may be associated with abnormally increased width between the two pubic bones, which may be as much as 35 mm (Scriven et al 1995). However the intensity of pain is not always relative to the size of the gap (Bjorklund et al 2000,

Snow & Neubert 1997) nor does the size of the gap predict outcome (Scriven et al 1995). This condition used to be referred to as diastasis of the symphysis pubis, but the term symphysis pubis dysfunction is more accurate and is widely used in current literature. The condition occurs in later pregnancy, occasionally during labour and rarely 24–36 hours postpartum. The latter is thought to be caused by an inflammatory process that takes time to manifest (Driessen 1987).

The function of the symphysis pubis joint is to complete the bony pelvic ring (see Figure 1.1) and transmit weight through the legs in an upright position. If the joint is not functioning correctly there will be abnormal function/stability of the pelvis which, coupled with mechanical changes taking place, severely affects gait – a gliding action taking place at the symphysis pubis joint on weight-bearing. This is extremely painful and produces a typical waddling gait.

The incidence is very difficult to quantify as the condition is under-recognised and under-diagnosed (Scriven et al 1995). Physiotherapists who have been working in the antenatal field for a number of years claim the incidence has risen over the last 10–15 years (personal communication). Snow and Neubert (1997) reported an incidence of approximately 1:569 after surveying 5121 women over a two-year period, Scriven et al (1995) found 1:800 whilst MacLennan & MacLennan (1997) stated that nearly one third of women they surveyed postnatally claimed they had experienced symphysis pubis pain during their pregnancies.

Symptoms include pain of varying intensity over the symphysis, radiating into the groin (uni/bilaterally) and sometimes into the medial aspect of the thigh. It may be associated with back and/or sacroiliac pain and is very much worse on weight-bearing, for example, walking or standing on one leg. Changing position exacerbates the pain, particularly turning in bed, getting out of bed or out of a car. Gait will be waddling or shuffling and climbing stairs may be impossible. On palpation, which should be performed very gently, there is often acute tenderness over the joint. Hip abduction may be very limited due to the pain and the woman's daily activities may be severely compromised (see Box 3.3).

Box 3.3 Characteristics of SPD

- pain over the pubis and medial aspect of the thigh often associated with low back pain and/or sacroiliac pain
- pain worse when standing on one leg
- grinding in the joint felt on movement and sometimes heard
- waddling gait pattern
- limited and painful abduction of the hips
- severe tenderness on palpation of the symphysis pubis joint.

There are implications for labour in those presenting antepartum. The range of pain-free abduction of the hips during pregnancy should be measured and documented in the notes so that this measurement is not exceeded during labour. Alternative positions for delivery, for example, side lying, high kneeling will be necessary to avoid undue hip abduction or in extreme cases an elective caesarean section will be necessary (Fry 1999). If the lithotomy position is unavoidable, care should be taken to ensure both legs are raised simultaneously to avoid disruption of the symphysis. Epidural anaesthesia will mask the pain and should be used with caution.

Kristiansson et al (1996) suggested the cause of SPD is ligament/joint laxity as a result of the effect of relaxin but serum relaxin levels were not found to be higher in women suffering from SPD (Bjorklund et al 2000).

Treatment during pregnancy

- referral to a women's health physiotherapist
- firm support around the level of the greater trochanters of the hip and the symphysis pubis, for example, trochanteric belt, sacroiliac support or three layers of tubigrip
- pain relief
- walking aids, for example, elbow crutches or zimmer frame if necessary
- advice re back care, activities of daily living, adequate rest
- correction of muscle imbalance
- measurement of pain-free range of abduction and documentation in notes for labour.

During labour/delivery

- all staff to be aware of the woman's condition to ensure best handling
- prevention of undue abduction beyond pain-free range
- avoidance of lithotomy position if possible, but movement of both legs must be simultaneous if lithotomy position is unavoidable
- side-lying or kneeling for delivery
- LSCS if very severe
- **NB** epidural/spinal will mask pain.

After delivery

- bed rest for as long as is necessary
- adequate pain relief
- complete mother and baby care may need to be provided

- referral to women's health physiotherapist for appropriate abdominal exercises
- circulatory exercises
- gradual mobilisation when pain less acute
- appropriate aids
- referral to occupational therapist, social services, health visitor etc. if necessary.

Mason & Pearson (2000) suggested it is necessary to raise the profile of SPD among the medical and midwifery professions to ensure that women suffering from the condition are treated with sympathy and receive appropriate advice. They recommended that all women are referred to a women's health physiotherapist.

Guidelines for the management of SPD have been produced by the Association of Chartered Physiotherapists in Women's Health (ACPWH 2000).

Box 3.4 summarises advice that can be given to women suffering from SPD.

Box 3.4   Advice for women suffering from SPD

- ask to be referred to a women's health physiotherapist
- rest as much as possible
- sleep on side with pillow between legs to separate the knees in line with hips
- avoid weight-bearing activities where possible, for example, climbing stairs, lifting, shopping
- avoid separating the hips and knees when getting out of bed
- keep knees pressed together when getting in/out of a car
- avoid breast stroke if swimming
- do not stand on one leg to put on trousers or tights
- avoid squatting positions/activities
- ensure hips are not unduly abducted during labour
- delivery in side-lying or high kneeling
- be aware that epidural anaesthesia will mask the pain

DIASTASIS RECTI

Diastasis recti is a separation of the muscle bellies of rectus abdominis of more than 2.5 cm at a level just above the umbilicus (Noble 1995) as a result of hormonal influence on the linea alba and mechanical stretching of the abdominal wall (see Figure 3.1). The pyrimidalis muscle helps to support the linea alba and Boissonault & Kotarinos (1988) suggested that its absence in some women may predispose them to a diastasis. The separation can occur towards the end of pregnancy (Hsia & Jones 2000)

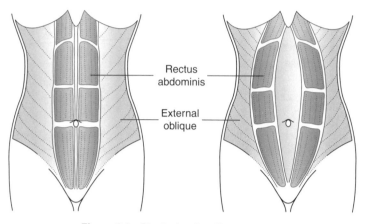

Rectus
abdominis

External
oblique

Figure 3.1   Diastasis of recti postpartum.

or occasionally occurs during labour especially if there has been prolonged breath-holding with pushing during the second stage (Noble 1995).
After delivery there will be some increase in the width between the rectus
bellies in all women. It is more common with multiple pregnancies, large
babies, polyhydramnios, weak abdominal muscles and poor posture, but
may appear for seemingly no apparent reason in slim, fit women. It is
thought that this might be due to some altered collagen make up which
can be familial and would explain the fact that some women and their
daughters experience diastasis without having any of the above criteria.
The incidence of diastasis greater than 2.5 cms is not widely reported but
Boissonault & Blashak (1988) claimed it to be 66%.

During pregnancy it is difficult to assess diastasis, which is characterised by doming of the abdominals on attempting to sit up from lying.
Doming will also occur postnatally on the same activity. In severe cases,
where the gap may be as much as 10 cms or even more, the abdomen will
resemble a whirlpool and the woman will complain of constant backache
as the abdominal muscles are no longer supporting the spine or pelvis. It
can be a frightening condition as the pulsating intestines may be visible
and the woman may feel that they may protrude even further on standing.
The largest reported distances between the muscle bellies appear to be
23 cms (Thornton & Thornton 1993). Normally a gap of 3–4 cms will
resolve over a week or two after appropriate abdominal exercise (see
below). However, Hsia & Jones (2000) found increased distances were still
present at 12 weeks post delivery whilst Thornton's diastasis did not fully
close until six months postpartum.

All women should have a rectus check postnatally to assess the distance
between the muscle bellies. This can be performed by the midwife or by

the woman herself or her partner. It is a simple procedure for the midwife to carry out after she has checked the fundus on the third or fourth day postpartum or seventh day post-caesarean delivery, and this check should be incorporated into standard postnatal practice.

Rectus check

The woman should lie on her back with one pillow under her head, knees bent up and feet flat on the bed. With one or two of the midwife's fingers pressed widthways into the abdomen either just above or below the umbilicus, the mother is asked to lift her head and shoulders off the pillow towards her knees. The rectus muscles should be felt taut either side of the finger(s) if there is no undue diastasis. If the rectus bellies cannot be felt, then 3 or even 4 fingers are inserted and the procedure repeated. The width of the fingers used can be measured with a tape and documented. Up to 2.5 cm (two slim fingers) width between the rectus muscles is considered acceptable. If the gap is greater than this, rotational activities should not be performed as the stress on the linea alba may increase the separation (see Ch. 8). Advice on the correct way to perform daily activities, especially getting up from the supine position, and progression of exercises should be given (see Ch. 9).

Subsequent pregnancies will increase the diastasis (Thornton & Thornton 1993) and women should be advised to wear some form of support for the abdominal muscles in any future pregnancy if an undue diastasis was reported in a previous pregnancy.

Treatment:

- rectus check to assess distance between rectus muscle bellies
- support in the form of tubigrip (double thickness if necessary) from xiphisternum to below buttocks
- transversus and pelvic floor exercises as often as possible in all positions except prone-kneeling
- ensure the woman does not perform curl-ups or sit-ups
- advice re activities of daily living – especially the avoidance of any activity which causes doming of the abdomen
- follow-up assessments by a women's health physiotherapist as long as is necessary
- advice on progression of exercises when gap has reduced
- advice re support during subsequent pregnancies.

Box 3.5 summarises advice that can be given to women suffering from diastasis of the recti.

Box 3.5 Advice for women suffering from diastasis recti

- ask for an assessment of the gap between the rectus muscle bellies
- perform transversus contractions as often as possible in all positions except prone kneeling
- avoid curl-ups and sit-ups
- wear tubigrip (double if getting backache) from the level of the bra to below the buttocks
- when getting out of bed always bend knees and roll over onto side keeping shoulders in line with knees, do not attempt to sit up forwards from lying supine
- brace abdominal and pelvic floor muscles before performing any activities
- avoid any activities/exercises which involve twisting until the gap has reduced to 2 cms
- avoid any activitiy which causes the abdomen to dome
- ask for follow up assessment from women's health physiotherapist
- wear some support during any subsequent pregnancy.

PREGNANCY-ASSOCIATED OSTEOPOROSIS (PAO)

This is a condition which may present in the third trimester of pregnancy or postnatally. There are no precise criteria for establishing the diagnosis of pregnancy-associated osteoporosis which is based on the historical progression of events in relation to pregnancy in the absence of other underlying causes and supported by radiological evidence of fracture and/or osteopenia (Dunne et al 1993). The presence of osteoporosis is determined by using dual energy X-ray absorptiometry (DEXA) scanning which is safe to use in pregnancy. Readings are compared to the young adult mean value. Over 2.5 standard deviations (SD) below the young adult mean is classed as osteoporosis (DOH 1994) whilst the term osteopenia is used to describe a reduction in bone mass without the presence of a fracture (Compston 1993) and is defined by the DOH as more than 1 SD but less than 2.5 SD below the young adult mean value.

Little literature on the subject is available, but what has been published highlights the lack of early recognition of the disease, and difficulty and delay in diagnosis, particularly during pregnancy. Dunne et al (1993), Funk et al (1995) and Smith et al (1995) all stated that the condition is under-diagnosed and poorly understood, whilst a survey of health professionals revealed a significant lack of knowledge of the condition amongst those working with pregnant/postnatal women (Brayshaw 1999).

PAO is characterised by pain, vertebral and hip fractures and disability. The condition tends to affect the older woman aged 27+ particularly those who sustain vertebral fractures. Disabilities include being unable to walk, inability to lift or feed the baby postnatally, reduced height and poor posture (Brayshaw 2002). (See Box 3.6).

Box 3.6   Characteristics of PAO

- pain in lower thoracic and/or upper lumbar spine or hips
- sudden spasms either side of spine
- fracture of the vertebrae, hip, ribs
- reduced mobility, inability to walk if hip fracture
- inability to lift, feed or care for baby if vertebral fractures
- poor posture
- reduced height if vertebral fractures.

It is important to obtain a diagnosis as early as possible so some fractures may be avoided. A caesarean section might prevent a fracture occurring during a vaginal delivery in the hip of an osteoporotic woman. If women were aware of their PAO, they would be able to make a decision about breastfeeding as it is known that lactation demands extra calcium requirements compared to pregnancy (Smith & Phillips 1998). Dunne et al (1993) advised cessation of lactation and Smith & Phillips (1998) stated that it is contraindicated in women with PAO as lactation maintains a low bone density. Women would be advised to avoid the weight bearing/lifting that might result in fractures.

Many causes of PAO have been postulated but no one factor has been identified. However there appears to be a genetic link as the parents of women with PAO had more unexplained fractures than those of controls (Dunne et al 1993), and the teenage daughters of two PAO sufferers studied by Carbone et al (1995) showed osteopenia of the hips on scanning.

PELVIC FLOOR DYSFUNCTION

Pelvic floor dysfunction may result in urinary or faecal incontinence.

Urinary incontinence

This is the complaint of involuntary leakage of urine (ICS 2002). The most common urinary problem in pregnancy and postpartum is stress incontinence. The International Continence Society (ICS) defines stress urinary incontinence as the complaint of involuntary leakage on effort or exertion, or on sneezing or coughing (ICS 2002). The pelvic floor muscles play a large part in maintaining the urethral pressure when there is a sudden rise in intra-abdominal pressure during stressful events. Normally the urethral pressure remains higher than the intra-abdominal pressure – maintaining continence – but if the pelvic floor muscles are weak the urethral pressure is not maintained and leaking results. The prevalence of stress incontinence in later pregnancy has been documented as 40% (Marshall et al 1996), 42% (Mørkved & Bø 1999) whilst Jolleys (1990) reported that 50% of primigravid women suffered, with a higher percentage still in multigravid women.

In many cases stress incontinence experienced during pregnancy reduces after delivery, but Wilson et al (1996) and Mørkved & Bø (1999) reported prevalences of 35% after childbirth whilst Marshall et al (1996) claimed that 59% of Irish women surveyed suffered some degree of leaking after birth with one third of these still leaking after nine months.

Reilly et al (2002) found that supervised antenatal pelvic floor exercises were effective in reducing the risk of postpartum stress incontinence in primigravid women. Bø (1995) reviewed studies investigating the effects of pelvic floor exercises for the treatment of stress incontinence and concluded that they are effective (up to 70% cure) and cost-effective when properly taught after an individual assessment. However she found no value in written or verbal instruction without a prior assessment of the pelvic floor muscles. Women need to have regular follow-ups for up to six months. Mørkved & Bø (1997) found that 66% of women were cured after an eight-week course of intensive pelvic floor exercises carried out between eight and 16 weeks postpartum. In a follow-up study they found that these women were still continent one year later (Mørkved & Bø 2000). They concluded that the specially-designed course of pelvic floor exercises were effective in increasing pelvic floor muscle strength and reducing urinary incontinence. Hay-Smith et al (2001) concurred with this finding in relation to stress incontinence and mixed incontinence.

Other types of incontinence that may affect postnatal women include frequency, urgency and urge incontinence. Frequency is described as the need to void urine more than eight times a day. This can be helped by pelvic floor exercises and bladder training. Urgency is defined as the complaint of a sudden compelling desire to pass urine, which is difficult to defer, whilst urge incontinence is the complaint of involuntary leakage accompanied by or immediately preceded by urgency (ICS 2002). It is caused by instability of the detrusor muscle of the bladder which contracts before the bladder is full.

NB It is extremely important that midwives monitor the urine output of women who have undergone epidural anaesthesia during childbirth. There may be delayed sensation for some time after the epidural and lack of awareness of the need to pass urine. This could lead to overstretching of the bladder and permanent bladder dysfunction.

Treatment

Antenatally, women should be taught and encouraged to practice pelvic floor and transversus exercises as often as possible (see Ch. 4) and to brace these muscles together with transversus when performing stressful activities.

Postnatally women should be encouraged to practise pelvic floor and transversus exercises immediately after birth and to continue for at least three months. Women who continue to suffer should be referred to a women's health physiotherapist who will assess their pelvic floor effectiveness and prescribe specific retraining programmes which may include biofeedback and stimulation if appropriate.

Faecal incontinence

This is a very distressing problem, which fortunately is very much less common than urinary incontinence. It is probably caused by the tearing or stretching of the anal sphincter or actual damage to the pelvic floor nerve supply during childbirth (Snooks et al 1985). Swash (1993) claimed that childbirth is responsible for most cases of faecal incontinence occurring in women and MacArthur et al (2001) found that women delivered by forceps had almost twice the risk of developing faecal incontinence. Depending on the severity of nerve damage, function may not be restored for several weeks and, in some cases, impairment may be permanent. Sultan et al (1993) found anal sphincter damage more likely in primigravid women and that 35% of the women they followed up still suffered from faecal incontinence 16 months after childbirth.

Treatment

Women with problems should be referred to a women's health physiotherapist for specialist assessment and treatment.

Prolapse

Genital prolapse is associated with vaginal deliveries (Wilson et al 1996), which may cause stretching and damage to the pelvic fascia and nerves. A uterine prolapse is a descent of the uterus, a cystocoele is a prolapse of the bladder into the vagina, whilst a rectocoele is a prolapse of the rectum into the vagina (Thakar & Stanton 2002). Women will complain of a feeling of something dropping down, especially when standing, backache and a dragging sensation.

Treatment

Minor prolapses may be helped by the practice of pelvic floor exercises and by bracing the pelvic floor and transversus before any stressful event such as coughing or lifting. A women's health physiotherapist will be able to assess and treat women presenting with this problem.

REFERENCES

ACPWH 2000 SPD Guidelines. Chartered Society of Physiotherapy, London

Bjorklund K, Bergstrom S, Nordstrom M L et al 2000 Symphyseal distention in relation to serum relaxin levels and pelvic pain in pregnancy. Acta Obstetrica Gynaecologica Scandinavica 79(4):269–275

Boissonault J S, Blaschak M J 1988 Incidence of diastasis recti abdominis during the childbearing year. Physical Therapy 68:1082–1086

Boissonault J S, Kotarinos R K 1988 Diastasis recti. In: Wilder E (ed) Obstetrics and Gynecological Physical Therapy. Churchill Livingstone, New York pp 63–82

Brayshaw E M 1999 An investigation into the current level of knowledge and awareness of pregnancy-associated osteoporosis amongst health professionals. Journal of the Chartered Physiotherapists in Women's Health 84:31

Brayshaw E 2002 Pregnancy-associated osteoporosis. Journal of the Chartered Physiotherapists in Women's Health 91:3–9

Breen T, Ransil B, Groves P et al 1994 Factors associated with back pain after childbirth. Anaesthesiology 81:29–34

Bø K 1995 Pelvic floor muscle exercise for the treatment of stress urinary incontinence: an exercise physiology perspective. International Urogynecology Journal 6:282–291

Bullock-Saxton J 1998 Musculoskeletal changes in the perinatal period. In: Sapsford R, Bullock-Saxton J, Markwell S (eds) Women's Health. W B Saunders, London

Butler R, Fuller J 1998 Back pain following epidural anaesthesia in labour. Canadian Journal of Anaesthesiology 45(8):724–728

Carbone L D, Palmieri G M A, Graves S C et al 1995 Osteoporosis in pregnancy: Long-term follow up of patients and their offspring. Obstetrics & Gynecology 86:664–666

Compston J 1993 Osteoporosis. In: Campbell G, Compston J, Crisp A (eds) The Management of Common Metabolic Bone Disorders. Cambridge University Press, Cambridge

Damen L, Buyruk H M, Guler-Usal F et al 2001 Pelvic pain during pregnancy is associated with asymmetric laxity of the sacroiliac joints. Acta Obstetrica Gynaecologica Scandinavica 80(11):1019–1024

Department of Health 1994 Advisory group on osteoporosis report. DOH

Driessen F 1987 Postpartum pelvic arthropathy with unusual features. British Journal of Obstetrics and Gynaecology 94:870–872

Dunne F, Walters B, Marshall T et al 1993 Pregnancy-associated osteoporosis. Clinical Endocrinology 39:487–490

Fry D 1999 Perinatal symphysis pubis dysfunction: a review of the literature. Journal of the Association of Chartered Physiotherapists in Women's Health 83:11–18

Funk J L, Shoback M, Genant K H 1995 Transient osteoporosis of the hip in pregnancy: natural history of changes in bone mineral density. Clinical Endocrinology 43:373–382

Hay-Smith E J, Bo Berghams L C, Hendricks H J et al (2001) Pelvic floor muscle training for urinary incontinence in women. Cochrane Database Systematic Revue (1):CD001407

Hsia M, Jones S 2000 Natural resolution of rectus abdominis diastasis. Two single case studies. Australian Journal of Physiotherapy 46:301–307

International Continence Society (2002) The Standardisation of Terminology in Lower Urinary Tract Function: Report from the Standardisation Sub-committee of the International Continence Society

Jolleys J V 1990 The reported prevalence of urinary symptoms in women in one rural practice. British Journal of General Practice 40:335–337

Kristiansson P, Svardsudd K, von Schoultz B 1996 Serum relaxin, symphyseal pain, and back pain during pregnancy. American Journal of Obstetrics and Gynecology 175(5):1342–1347

MacArthur C, Lewis W, Knox E G et al 1990 Epidural anaesthesia and longterm backache after childbirth. British Medical Journal 301:9–12

MacArthur C, Glazener C M A, Wilson P D et al 2001 Obstetric practice and faecal incontinence three months after delivery. British Journal of Obstetrics and Gynaecology 108:678–683

McEvoy A, Howlett M, Langton A et al 2001 Back pain during pregnancy in Irish women. Journal of the Association of Chartered Physiotherapists in Women's Health 89:6–9

MacLennan A H & MacLennan S C 1997 Symptom-giving pelvic girdle relaxation of pregnancy, postnatal pelvic joint syndrome and developmental dysplasia of the hip. Acta Obstetrica Gynecologica Scandinavica 76:760–764

Mantle J 1994 Back pain in the childbearing year. In: Bayling J D, Palastanga N (eds) Grieve's Modern Manual Therapy 2nd edn Churchill Livingstone, Edinburgh

Marshall K, Totterdal D, McConnell V et al 1996 Urinary incontinence and constipation during pregnancy and after childbirth. Physiotherapy 82(2):98–103

Mason G, Pearson A 2000 Symphysis pubis dysfunction. Journal of the Association of Chartered Physiotherapists in Women's Health 87:3–4

Mørkved S, Bø K 1997 The effect of postpartum pelvic floor exercise in the prevention and treatment of urinary incontinence. International Urogynecological Journal 8:217–222

Mørkved S, Bø K 1999 Prevalence of urinary incontinence during pregnancy and postpartum. International Urogynecological Journal 10:394–398

Mørkved S, Bø K 2000 Effect of postpartum pelvic floor muscle training in prevention and treatment of urinary incontinence: a one-year follow up. British Journal of Obstetrics & Gynaecology 107:1022–1028

Noble E 1995 Essential Exercises for the Childbearing Year. New Life Images, New York

Östgaard H C (1995) Back and posterior pelvic pain in relation to pregnancy. In: Vleeming A, Mooney V, Dorman T et al (eds) The integral function of the lumbar spine and sacroiliac joint. Second Interdisciplinary World Congress on Low Back Pain, San Diego, pp 185–188

Östgaard H C, Andersson G B I 1991 Previous back pain and risk of developing back pain in a future pregnancy 16(4):432–436

Östgaard H C, Andersson G B I 1992 Postpartum low back pain. Spine 17(1):53–55

Östgaard H C, Andersson G B I, Karlsson K 1991 Prevalence of back pain in pregnancy. Spine 16:549–552

Reilly E T, Freeman R M, Waterfield M R et al 2002 Prevention of postpartum stress incontinence in primigravidae with increased bladder neck mobility: a randomised control trial of antenatal pelvic floor exercises. British Journal of Obstetrics and Gynaecology 109(1):68–76

Rungee M J L (1993) Low back pain during a pregnancy. Orthopaedics 16:1339–1344

Russell R, Groves P, Taub N et al 1993 Assessing long term backache after childbirth. British Medical Journal 306:1299–1303

Scriven M W, Jones D A, McKnight L 1995 The importance of pubic pain following childbirth: a clinical and ultrasonographic study of diastasis of the pubic symphysis. Journal of the Royal Society of Medicine 88:28–30

Smith R, Athanasou N A, Ostlere S J et al 1995 Pregnancy-associated osteoporosis. Quarterly Journal of Medicine 88:865–878

Smith R, Phillips A J 1998 Osteoporosis during pregnancy and its management. Scandinavian Journal of Rheumatology Supplement 107:66–67

Snooks S J, Henry M M, Swash M 1985 Faecal incontinence due to external sphincter division in childbirth is associated with damage to innervation of the pelvic floor musculature. A double pathology. British Journal of Obstetrics and Gynaecology 92:824–828

Snow R E, Neubert A G 1997 Peripartum pubic symphysis separation: a case series and review of the literature. Obstetrical and Gynecological Survey 52(7): 438–443

Sultan A H, Kamm M A, Hudson C H et al 1993 Anal sphincter disruption during vaginal delivery. New England Journal of Medicine 329(26):1905–1911

Swash M 1993 Faecal incontinence, childbirth is responsible for most cases. British Medical Journal 307:636–637

Thakar R, Stanton S 2002 Management of genital prolapse. British Medical Journal 324(7348):1258–1262

Thornton S I, Thornton S J 1993 Management of gross divarification of the recti abdominis in pregnancy and labour. Physiotherapy 79:457–458

Wilson P D, Herbison R M, Herbison G P 1996 Obstetric practice and the prevalence of urinary incontinence three months after delivery. British Journal of Obstetrics and Gynaecology 103:154–161

Young G, Jewell D 2000 Interventions for preventing and treating backache in pregnancy. Cochrane Database Systematic Review 2000(2) CD001139

4

Antenatal exercises and advice

Basic antenatal
  exercises 42
  Circulatory exercises 42
  Pelvic floor exercises 44
  Abdominal exercises 45
Backcare in pregnancy 47
  Sitting 48
  Standing 49

Lying 50
Lifting 52
Household activities 53
Additional exercises 54
  Stretching exercises 54
  General exercise 55
Exercises to avoid 55
References 56

This chapter covers the input that would normally be introduced by a women's health physiotherapist if there is one in the team. The specific antenatal exercises and advice may be incorporated into a scheme of preparation for parenthood classes in the hospital or community setting. They may also be useful for the midwife on a one-to-one basis.

In her book, Safe Childbirth (1937), Dr Kathleen Vaughan described how her work with pregnant women who had led sedentary, inactive lives had shown that they frequently had difficult labours and deliveries. She recounted that for women of the Outer Hebrides who led laborious but healthy lives, and Kashmiri boatwomen and peasants, labour was easier. The way women used their bodies in everyday life had an important influence before, during and after childbirth.

Many exercise programmes have been devised over the years (Balaskas & Balaskas 1979; Dale & Roeber 1982; Heardman 1948; McLaren 1978; Madders 1965; Noble 1978; Randell 1948; Wright 1964). Despite the trend which some women follow towards continuing their chosen sport or activity into the later stages of their pregnancy, life for many is far less physically demanding than in the forties and fifties. Cars, washing machines and other present-day appliances have made life much easier physically.

It is important for a woman to maintain or improve her physical condition if she is to remain at her best throughout pregnancy and overcome the stresses placed upon her body by the development of the baby. Women who exercise have shorter labours with less intervention and a speedy recovery after the birth (Clapp 2000). Advice should be offered about sport and other activities. Swimming and walking should be encouraged to help maintain cardiovascular and respiratory fitness, general body muscle tone and relieve tension. The continuation of participation in competitive contact sports should be discouraged, and it is also inadvisable to start any new strenuous activity during pregnancy. However, for those women who wish to continue some fairly vigorous activity, antenatal aerobic and/or aquanatal sessions would be a sensible alternative, provided these were led by fully qualified instructors (see Ch. 12). Moderate exercise has become the recommended formula for most mothers-to-be. Ideally women should increase their fitness prior to pregnancy.

The contents of this chapter will help women to address the physiological effects of pregnancy (particularly those affecting the musculoskeletal system), to help them to cope with the minor stresses and strains of pregnancy, and to prepare them for labour and the immediate postnatal period. The aim is to prevent any short or long-term problems that could arise as the result of the changes taking place during the childbearing year. Chapter 12 analyses other forms of exercise that would complement the antenatal exercises described here.

Antenatal classes are the ideal forum to teach exercises but the women need to be encouraged to practise them at home or at work whenever possible and to bring in the transversus and pelvic floor muscles during everyday functional activities.

BASIC ANTENATAL EXERCISES

Circulatory exercises

Circulatory exercises should be practised frequently, particularly in the early morning and late evening. They should be performed in a half-lying or sitting position with the legs elevated and are intended to maintain and improve the circulation. Vigorous movements of the feet will assist venous return and minimise varicosities, swelling of the ankles and cramp (Figure 4.1).

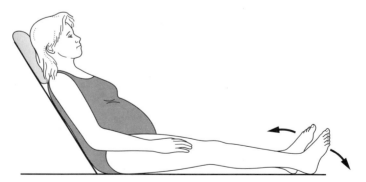

Figure 4.1   Foot exercises.

Foot exercises

- Sit or lie at an angle of 45 degrees (half-lying) with the back against a wedge and pillows, the legs supported and the knees straight. Bend and stretch the ankles briskly at least 12 times, emphasising dorsiflexion rather than plantar flexion to avoid cramp. Keeping the knees and hips still, circle both ankles in as large a circle as possible at least 12 times in each direction.

Leg-tightening

- Sit or lie (half-lying) in the same position as above. Pull both feet upwards at the ankle and press the back of the knees down onto the support. Hold this position for a count of 5, breathing normally, then relax. Repeat 10 times.

A pregnant woman should be advised to avoid prolonged standing, and sitting or lying with her legs crossed. She should be encouraged to sit with her feet raised on a low stool. If oedema is present, she could lie at an angle of 45 degrees with her legs raised a little higher than her hips (see Figure 4.2).

It is important to retain a wide angle at the groin in order to prevent compression, which could cause circulatory stasis. A pillow under the bottom of the mattress will elevate her feet when sleeping. Sitting instead of standing must be encouraged whilst doing household chores such as ironing, peeling vegetables etc. The woman should be reminded that walking will aid her circulation especially the deep venous blood flow. She should be advised to wear good supporting footwear and avoid high heels, which might cause injury through instability. If a woman has always worn high heels then she should not wear completely flat shoes but something with a lower heel and a broader base.

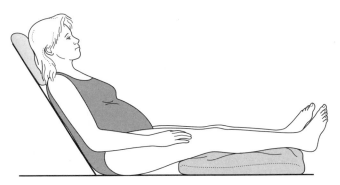

Figure 4.2 Legs elevated in a half-lying position.

Pelvic floor exercises

Pelvic-floor exercises should receive top priority in any programme of physical exercise during pregnancy. Muscles toned antenatally will be able to cope with the stresses and strains put on them by pregnancy and to give extra support to the fascial layer which is relaxing under the influence of relaxin. The woman will also understand how to re-educate them after delivery to help to prevent any long-term urinary problems or prolapse. Pelvic-floor exercises should be taught, even late in pregnancy. Healthy, exercised muscles stretch and recoil more easily, which can facilitate delivery. It has been shown that pelvic floor muscles are stronger postnatally in women who exercised during pregnancy than in those who did not (Nielsen, 1988) and that antenatal pelvic floor exercises reduced the risk of postpartum stress incontinence in primigravidae (Reilly et al 2002). It has also been highlighted that the pelvic floor muscles play a part in maintaining the stability of the pelvis (see Ch. 2).

Ideally women will have been introduced to pelvic floor exercises before pregnancy, but many women will not have performed them. The exercise should be started as early as possible in pregnancy at an early bird class if one is available (see Ch. 11). Before the exercise is taught, the relevant anatomy and the importance of these muscles must be explained in simple terms. A model pelvis and drawings will be helpful.

The pelvic floor exercise

The pelvic floor exercise can be practised in any comfortable position as long as the legs are slightly apart, not crossed.

* Squeeze the back passage as though preventing a bowel action, squeeze the middle and front passages too as though preventing the flow of urine, then lift up all three passages inside. Hold strongly for as long as possible up to 10 seconds, breathing normally throughout. Relax and rest for 3 seconds. Repeat slowly as many times as you can, up to a maximum of 10. Repeat the exercise, this time lifting up and letting go more quickly up to 10 times without holding the contraction. Avoid tightening the buttocks and thigh muscles.

To define your personal programme for your pelvic floor, remember the number of seconds for which you can hold the contraction and the number times you can repeat the exercise before the muscle becomes tired. Aim to try to improve both numbers up to 10 times 10 over the weeks.

By exercising these muscles slowly and quickly, both the slow-twitch (type I) and fast-twitch (type II) muscle fibres will be activated (Gilpin et al 1989). A reliable schedule for the exercise may be provided by linking them to daily activities, for example washing up, after each bladder-emptying, or by displaying stickers around the house as reminders.

Time must be given in the session for questions and discussion to help the women to try out the exercise and to understand it thoroughly. Some may need further advice in order fully to appreciate the feeling and to be confident that they can contract the muscles. Chiarelli (1991) stated that it might prove dangerous to use the urine 'stop and start' mechanism as an exercise, as this practice is not good bladder-training. However, a midstream stop could be used as an occasional test, preferably on the second or subsequent voiding of the day. Another way to recognise the contractions might be by observation in a mirror when semi-squatting. Gripping the penis during intercourse, thus sharing the exercise with the partner, can have the benefit of feedback. Women should be advised to contract their pelvic floor before coughing, sneezing, laughing, lifting or squatting. The pelvic floor contraction can be combined with the transversus exercise (see below).

Abdominal exercises

Because of their attachment to the linea alba, exercises involving the oblique abdominals, for example, twisting or knee rolling, should be avoided during later pregnancy to avoid the risk of tearing the linea alba and causing diastasis of the rectus muscles (Noble 1995). However, it is very important to exercise the deep abdominal muscles during pregnancy. Transversus abdominis has been found to be the core stability muscle (Hodges 1999) and needs to work as efficiently as possible to help maintain the integrity of the pelvis. It has been shown that the transversus abdominis is much more important than rectus abdominis in preventing postural and back problems (Horsley 1998) and so should be the main muscle to exercise during pregnancy and postpartum. It has a high proportion of slow twitch type I fibres which respond to a gentle – not maximal – contraction. The transversus exercise can be performed in any position, for example, sitting, standing, high-kneeling, prone-kneeling or side-lying (see Ch. 10). Kneeling on all fours (see Figure 4.3) is usually a comfortable position to start to learn the exercise, which should then be practised in any functional position during the day.

Transversus exercise

- Keeping the spine in the mid position, breathe in then gently draw in the lower abdominal muscles on the outward breath and hold the contraction for up to 10 seconds whilst continuing to breathe normally, then relax slowly. Repeat up to 10 times.

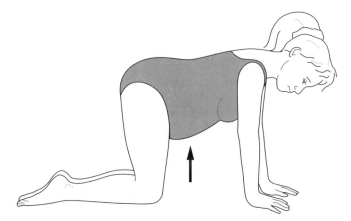

Figure 4.3 Transversus exercise in prone-kneeling.

Try to do this exercise often during the day whilst you are doing other activities.

Transversus and pelvic floor exercise

The actions of both the transversus and the pelvic floor muscles will be enhanced by combining the two exercises (Sapsford et al 2001). This may be done by working transversus then bringing in a pelvic floor contraction or vice versa. It is important to use this combined contraction to protect the spine and pelvic joints when performing functional activities such as moving and handling objects, changing positions, unavoidable standing.

As pregnancy progresses, the pelvic tilt alters putting a strain on the ligaments and joints of the lower back and pelvis which may lead to pain and discomfort. Pelvic tilting is a useful exercise to relieve back pain and stiffness, and promote good posture. Performed more quickly (pelvic rocking), the exercise helps to relieve backache in labour.

Pelvic tilting (rocking)

Lie at an angle of 45 degrees (half-lying) supported by a wedge and pillows, with the knees bent and the feet flat on the surface (Figure 4.4).

- Pull in the abdominal muscles, tighten the muscles of the buttocks and press the small of the back down onto the support. Hold the position for a count of 5, breathing normally, then relax. Repeat up to 10 times.

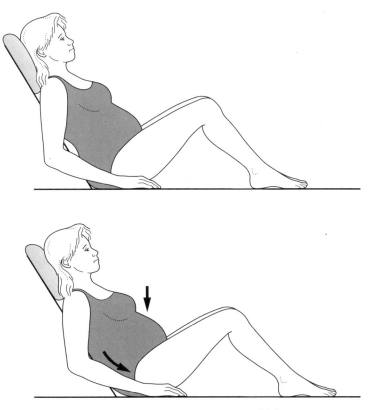

Figure 4.4   Pelvic tilting exercise in half-lying.

The exercise may also be performed more rhythmically (pelvic rocking) to help relieve any tension and postural backache whenever the need arises. Once mastered in this position, pelvic tilting or rocking can be encouraged in several positions, for example sitting, reverse sitting astride a chair, side-lying, standing, supported kneeling and prone kneeling (see Ch. 10).

BACKCARE IN PREGNANCY

The body, whether it is stationary or moving, should be respected at all times. However, this is especially important during pregnancy and for many months following delivery. During these times, the back and pelvic area are particularly vulnerable (see Ch. 2). To prevent long-term back problems and strain on stretched muscles, extra consideration must be given to the back when sitting, lifting, bending and moving, and during household and work-based activities. The midwife will need to explain the relevant anatomy and physiology to women and their partners and discuss possible problems. A model pelvis which has ligaments attached is very helpful to illustrate joints and vulnerable areas. In antenatal classes, small groups of women and partners can be asked to consider positions, movements and tasks that could lead to problems. This, followed by a whole-group feedback and discussion, is an interesting way of covering this topic. Heavy, strenuous work should be avoided. Rather than risking pain and tiredness, help should be requested. However, guidance and advice on how she might adapt and modify daily activities can allow the woman to continue many of her commitments well into pregnancy. She should be reminded to brace her transversus and pelvic floor muscles before undertaking any activities.

Sitting

Sitting is a commonly adopted position, so good posture and comfort are essential. A woman needs to be reminded to sit well back in her chair making sure that her lumbar spine is supported (see Figure 4.5). A small cushion or rolled towel may be needed to achieve this. The thighs should be supported by the chair, the feet resting flat on the floor. It may be necessary to have the feet raised on a small stool or cushion if they do not reach the floor comfortably. A chair with a high back would support the head and shoulders and the legs could be elevated on a foot stool. This would be an ideal position for relaxation practice. When getting up from the chair, transversus and the pelvic floor muscles should be activated.

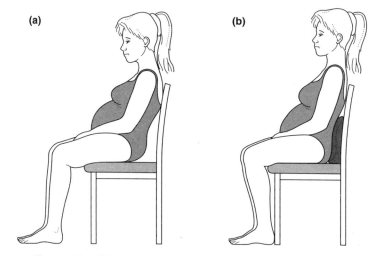

Figure 4.5 (a) Poor posture in sitting; (b) Good posture in sitting.

Standing

The aspects of good upright posture must be discussed. The woman needs to be encouraged to stand and walk tall, using transversus and the pelvic floor. The position of the head is important – it should be held high with the chin tucked in and with shoulders down and relaxed. It might be suggested that the woman imagines a thread pulling her up to the ceiling from the head – to think tall and stretch out the spine. Alternatively she could be asked to try to stretch between the hips and the ribs to make more room for the baby. This will lessen the curves and so reduce the muscular effort used during standing. In order to keep good balance, the feet should be apart with the body weight distributed evenly through both legs and down through the outer border of each foot (see Figure 4.6). Standing still for too long can lead to tiredness and strain. So it is better to walk around but it is important that all the points of good, upright posture should be maintained. The woman should listen to her body and not walk for too long as this can lead to discomfort.

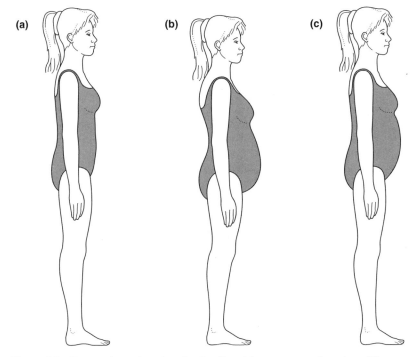

Figure 4.6 Poor and good posture in standing. (a) non-pregnant posture; (b) poor pregnant posture; (c) good pregnant posture.

Lying

Because of the risk of supine hypotension, lying flat on the back should be discouraged after the fourth month of pregnancy (see Ch. 2). If the supine position is used in early pregnancy, a pillow under the thighs gives extra comfort (see Figure 4.7). As pregnancy advances, the woman usually finds more difficulty in getting comfortable because of the increase in her size

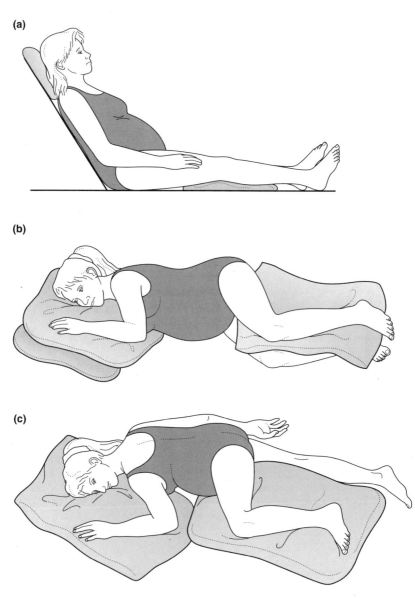

(a)

(b)

(c)

Figure 4.7   (a) Half-lying; (b) side lying; (c) three-quarters lying.

and weight. It is important that she alters her position and is well-supported giving equal pressure on all parts of the body in order to get rest and sleep and to prevent strain. For half-lying, extra pillows or a wedge will raise the head and shoulders enough and a pillow under the thighs will prevent stretch on the lower back and knees. Most women prefer side-lying with two pillows under the head and one under the top knee and thigh to prevent strain on the sacroiliac joint. A small cushion or rolled towel may add to comfort if placed under the waist or abdomen, especially if the mattress is not very firm. If side-lying is chosen, an extra pillow should be used to support the top forearm (Figure 4.7). Pain and strain at the symphysis pubis and sacroiliac joints can be minimised if the woman bends her knees up and keeps them pressed together when she turns over in bed.

Getting up from the bed or examination couch should be demonstrated to the group and practised. Both knees must be bent and kept together, the whole body rolled over to one side and then pushed up into the sitting position using the upper hand and lower elbow, with the legs now over the side of the bed. The woman slowly stands up, straightening her legs (see Figure 4.8).

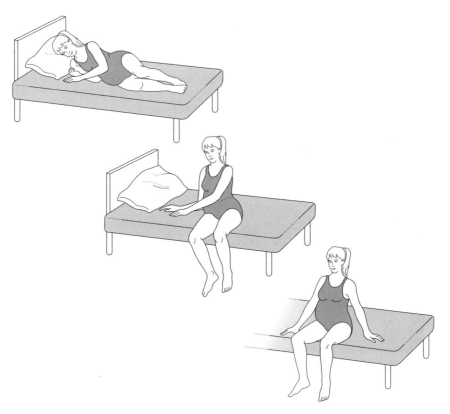

Figure 4.8 Getting up from lying.

This is done in reverse when getting onto a bed or couch. Midwives need to encourage this care in antenatal clinics, not only to protect the back, but also the linea alba. Trying to sit straight up forwards is similar to performing a sit-up exercise and must be discouraged. When rising from the floor, the woman should go over on her hands and knees and then push herself up onto one knee using the opposite arm for support. She then pushes herself up into the standing position by slowly straightening her legs. This again requires demonstration and practice.

Lifting

Heavy, difficult lifting should, whenever possible, be avoided during pregnancy. When having to lift, for example toddlers, the feet should be apart – one foot in front of the other – the hips and knees bent keeping the back straight, and the pelvic floor and transversus muscles should be tightened. Unless the thigh muscles are very strong, it places too much strain on the knee joints if women are advised to bend both knees to their full extent. The object to be lifted needs to be held close and central to the body, and the arms and legs used for lifting (see Figure 4.9).

This would be done in reverse to put down a heavy object. Twisting when lifting must be avoided and only when in the erect position should the feet be moved in the direction intended. If the woman is lifting a toddler, she could encourage him/her to stand on a chair or on the second or third step of the stairs so that she can avoid stooping to lift.

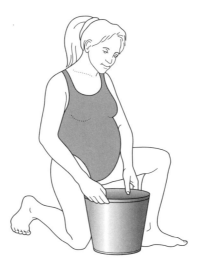

Figure 4.9 Correct lifting.

Household activities

Women can be advised to perform housework in an easy, rhythmical way – avoiding jerky movements, so putting less strain on the body and avoiding tiredness. Vacuuming must be performed in a straight line, avoiding twisting as this could stress the sacroiliac joints and the linea alba. Working levels need to be checked to maintain good posture – a high stool can prevent leaning and possible backache. Women can be encouraged to sit rather than stand for some tasks. Sitting down to do the ironing with the board lowered would be ideal but getting accustomed to this takes some practice! Alternatively, if ironing in the standing position is preferred, the height of the board should be such as to allow comfort with the feet apart and space to move rhythmically from side to side. When bathing toddlers, making beds, cleaning the bath or cuddling little ones, kneeling will prevent backache (see Figure 4.10). Some women will be able to use the squatting position, with one knee in front of the other, when getting down to low cupboards or drawers or to cuddle, again preventing lumbar strain; others will prefer to kneel to avoid stooping.

When shopping, women should keep the supermarket trolley close to the body and, ideally, load-carrying should be reduced to a minimum. If carrying the shopping, it can either be held close to the body or separated into two equal amounts for balanced transport (see Figure 4.11).

When getting into the car, sit first and then, tightening the transversus and pelvic floor muscles and keeping the knees together, bring the legs round into the car; this should be performed in reverse when getting out.

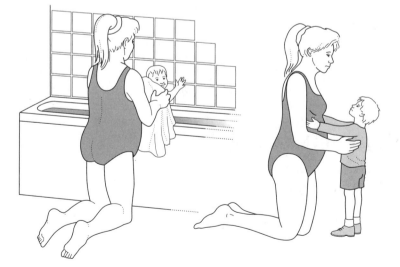

Figure 4.10 Kneeling to bath and cuddle toddler.

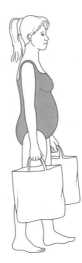

Figure 4.11   Carrying shopping.

When driving, the back needs to be well supported. Care should be taken, when putting on the seat belt and when reversing, to avoid twisting round in a jerky way.

Care of the back is an essential topic for inclusion in antenatal sessions with discussion and demonstrations. It is important to try·to prevent problems before they arise and cause pain. For this reason, consideration of baby equipment, and care in relation to backs and safety should be covered. It can be especially interesting for topics such as nappy-changing and bathing to be discussed with women when partners are present. They should realise that activities need to be stopped before pain is felt. Helping the women and partners to recognise what could cause this pain, so learning body-awareness, will prevent problems. They should be reminded that the more often a correct movement (for example, lifting) is performed, the more likely the performance will become an automatic, learned pattern of movement.

ADDITIONAL EXERCISES

Instructions for shoulder and arm exercises are included in Chapter 10 and may be incorporated into conventional preparation for parenthood classes.

Stretching exercises

The muscles and ligaments of the groin, hips and lower limbs (especially the adductors and calf muscles) will have shortened in many women, mainly due to our sedentary life style. Stretching exercises will help women to take up and hold various positions more comfortably during labour and delivery. The exercises prepare the women both physically and psychologically and encourage them to feel comfortable with wide-open legs, a position which they are not used to adopting (see Ch. 10).

General exercise

General exercise such as walking and swimming should be encouraged to maintain physical fitness and tone the muscles around the pelvis (see Ch. 12).

EXERCISES TO AVOID

Two commonly-practised 'abdominal exercises' are double-leg raising and sit-ups with straight legs (see Figure 4.12).

These are very high-risk exercises for anyone to perform and may result in compression injury to vertebral discs and muscle and ligament damage (Donovan et al 1988). There are added risks to the pregnant woman because of stretched muscles and lax ligaments (see Ch. 2).

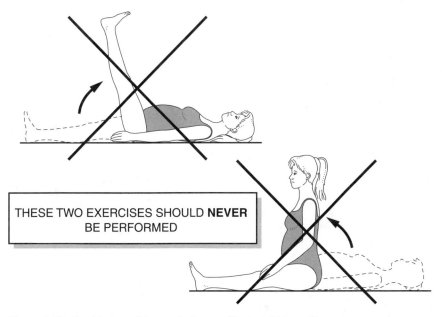

THESE TWO EXERCISES SHOULD **NEVER** BE PERFORMED

Figure 4.12 Double-leg raising and sit-ups with straight legs. These two exercises should *never* be practised but especially not during pregnancy.

REFERENCES

Balaskas A, Balaskas J 1979 New Life. Sidgwick and Jackson, London
Chiarelli P E 1991 Women's Waterworks: Curing Incontinence. Gore and Osment Publishing Pty Ltd. New South Wales
Clapp J F 3rd 2000 Exercise during pregnancy. A clinical update. Clinics in Sports Medicine (2):273–286
Dale B, Roeber J 1982 Exercises for Childbirth. Century Publishing, London
Donovan G, McNamara J, Gianoli P 1988 Exercise Danger. Wellness Australia Pty Ltd. Western Australia
Gilpin S A, Gosling J A, Smith A R B et al 1989 The pathogenesis of genitourinary prolapse and stress incontinence of urine. A histological and histochemical study. British Journal of Obstetrics and Gynaecology 96:15–23
Heardman H 1948 A Way to Natural Childbirth. E and S Livingstone, Edinburgh
Hodges P W 1999 Is there a role for transversus in lumbo-pelvic stability? Manual Therapy 4(2):74–86
Horsley K 1998 Fitness in the childbearing year. In: Sapsford R, Bullock-Saxton J, Markwell S (eds) Women's Health. W B Saunders, London
McLaren J 1978 Preparation for Parenthood. John Murray, London
Madders J 1965 Before and After Childbirth. E and S Livingstone, Edinburgh
Nielsen C A, Sigsgaard I, Olsen M et al 1988 Trainability of the pelvic floor. Acta Obstetrica Gynecologica Scandinavica 67:437–440
Noble E 1978 Essential Exercises for the Childbearing Year 1st edn. John Murray, London
Noble E 1995 Essential Exercises for the Childbearing Year 4th edn. New Life Images Harwich USA
Randell M 1948 Fearless Childbirth. Churchill, London
Reilly E T, Freeman R M, Waterfield M R et al 2002 Prevention of postpartum stress incontinence in primigravidae with increased bladder neck mobility: a randomized controlled trial of antenatal pelvic floor exercises. British Journal of Obstetrics and Gynaecology 109(1):68–76
Sapsford R R, Hodges P W, Richardson C A et al 2001 Co-activation of the abdominal and pelvic floor muscles during voluntary exercises. Neurourology and Urodynamics 20:31–42
Vaughan K 1937 Safe Childbirth. Ballière Tindall and Cox
Wright E 1964 The New Childbirth. Tandem, London

5

Stress and relaxation

What is stress? 57
Stress in Pregnancy 59
　How can we cope with
　　stress? 60
Relaxation techniques 60
　Progressive relaxation 60
　Physiological relaxation 61
　Touch 65

Massage 66
Aromatherapy 66
Imagery and suggestion 66
Hypnosis 66
Transcendental meditation (TSM) 67
Yoga 67
References 67
Further reading 67

This chapter includes the effects of stress on all of us in our everyday lives and also the additional stress that pregnancy brings. Methods of dealing with stress are discussed and the physiological method of relaxation for use during pregnancy, and labour in particular, is described in detail.

Relaxation is a topic included in most preparation for parenthood courses as women and partners request its inclusion and they are therefore interested and motivated. Most of us show some signs of tension when difficulties pile up. We feel tense, achy and tired and we even question whether we can cope. It is often a very insignificant incident which can turn out to be the last straw and which can finally 'break the camel's back'. We say that we are 'uptight' or under stress.

WHAT IS STRESS?

The stress of modern day living, a popular phrase today, may be brought about by any situation which gives rise to anxiety, uneasiness, irritation, fear, frustration or even anger. In biological language, stress means anything that creates a threat, whether real or imaginary, which might adversely impinge upon an organism.

The body prepares for 'fight or flight' whenever it seems to be threatened. This is a primitive animal instinct – an emergency reaction. However, in humans such reactions are produced not just when there is real danger, but also when there is no real threat to life at all. Unfortunately, it is this human inability to distinguish between the real and the imaginary threat, which can eventually lead to stress disorders. Some tension is necessary for performance but too much reduces achievement and leads to fatigue, pain and possibly illness. As soon as a threat is recognised, a reflex which

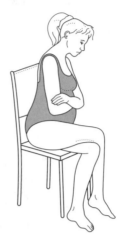

Figure 5.1 Stress position.

short-cuts the brain is triggered. Muscles immediately tense for action ready in the fight-flight response. We assume the common posture of tension. In sitting (see Figure 5.1):

1. the head comes forwards
2. the shoulders are elevated
3. the elbows are flexed and kept close to the body
4. the fists are clenched
5. the legs are crossed with feet dorsiflexed
6. the body is bent forwards and is usually rigid
7. the facial expression is often one of worry with the jaw clamped tightly shut.

This position of tension would be modified in standing or lying.

The danger message is received by the brain and internal responses are made. Dramatic changes in the working of the cardiovascular system become evident. The heart rate increases, the blood pressure rises and constriction of blood vessels in the skin and the digestive and reproductive systems results in diversion of blood to the brain, lungs and locomotor muscles. The respiratory system is also affected; breathing is either held on an inward gasp or becomes shallower and more rapid. The emphasis is on inspiration. Additionally, the mouth becomes dry, sweating increases and other more complicated changes occur (see Figure 5.2). When appropriate action has been taken and the danger is over, everything settles down to normal, relaxation takes place and no harm is done. It is when these normal and valuable reactions are prolonged, exaggerated and inappropriate that illness and disease can result.

Adopting the position of tension in itself causes increased tension and fatigue. Prolonged arousal can lead to others noticing the signs of strain

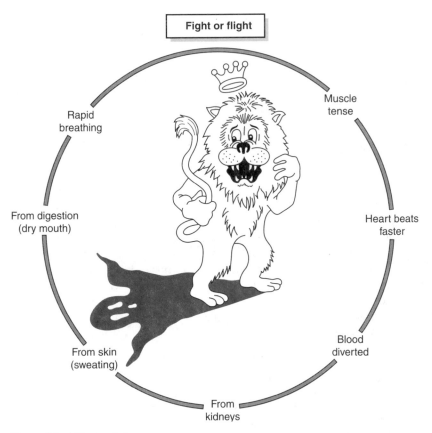

Figure 5.2 Effects of stress.

such as grumbling, irritability, decreased achievement at work (although more time spent there!), increased smoking and drinking and inadequate sleep. It is at this stage that the straw will 'break the camel's back'.

STRESS IN PREGNANCY

The American psychiatrists, Drs. Holmes and Rahe (1967), devised a scale of various stressful events, pregnancy being high on the scale. In pregnancy, the woman's body is in a different and changing physiological condition, which will affect not only her physical state but her psychological state too. She will have all the everyday stresses to which we are subjected plus the physical and emotional pressures that pregnancy brings. To mention but a few of these stresses:

1. was the baby planned?
2. will it be healthy?

3. what is the mother's work situation?
4. is she under stress to stay at work as long as possible and return to work afterwards?
5. is she provided with adequate finance?
6. has she a supportive partner?

She will also have the physical stresses of pregnancy to cope with:

1. is she exhausted and nauseous?
2. has she aching joints?
3. does she feel clumsy and less mobile?

Additionally, she may be anxious about labour and motherhood which will give rise to added tension. The pregnant woman also shares the physical effects of her emotions with the fetus. If her feelings of anxiety are increased, especially if they are prolonged and extreme, they may affect her baby. The increased chemicals and hormones produced by the anxiety state circulate in the body and can cross the placenta and reach the fetus (Madders, 1979). There may also be a relationship between a new baby's restlessness and extensive crying, and a mother's emotional distress. All the systems of the body are affected and the challenges these changes make on the pregnant woman should never be underestimated.

How can we cope with stress?

1. We can learn to understand ourselves, to realise how much we can put up with and to admit if we cannot cope.
2. We should take time out for hobbies and leisure activities.
3. We should, if possible, create some space for ourselves.
4. We should eat well, exercise and keep fit.

We should recognise that relaxation can be an efficient way of dealing with stress. A state of muscle relaxation is incompatible with that of anxiety. A relaxed person cannot be anxious, nor when anxious, can be truly relaxed (Woodrow 1988).

RELAXATION TECHNIQUES
Progressive relaxation

This was commonly called the contrast method and was taught in childbirth education classes. Dr Edmund Jacobsen outlined the technique, which involved alternately contracting and relaxing muscle groups progressively throughout the body (Jacobsen 1938). From this, the woman learned to recognise the difference between relaxation and tension.

Unfortunately, many using this method found that the body remained in a posture of tension, as those muscles that were tense were never lengthened – so the position of tension remained. Also, normal breathing was affected as breath-holding often took place as each muscle group was contracted.

Physiological relaxation

Physiological reciprocal relaxation is now the method more widely taught by women's health physiotherapists and midwives. It was developed by Laura Mitchell in 1987 and is a simple, exact technique. If one group of muscles is contracted, the opposite muscle group is stretched (relaxed). Clear orders are given to the opposite group of muscles to work and so the muscles that were tense are compelled to relax. This method is based on the physiological principle of reciprocal relaxation. Muscles move the joints into a position of ease; this will be a neutral position. In her book, *Simple Relaxation* (1987), Laura Mitchell points out that information about the state of relaxation or contraction of a muscle is not carried to the conscious brain – the brain only receives information about a muscle's movement. Proprioceptors in joints and muscle tendons, and receptors in the skin register the resulting position of ease and this is communicated to the brain where it is recorded in the cerebrum. Clear and concise instructions are given to each area of the body affected by stress. Three instructions are used in a fixed order throughout the body and they result in body awareness of the posture of ease for relaxation.

The sequence of instructions for each joint is:

1. **move** into the position opposite to that of stress
2. **stop** doing the movement
3. **check** the new position of the joint and, if applicable, the skin sensation.

Relaxation for the pregnant woman and partner may be practised in any comfortable, supported position – sitting (see Figure 5.3), side-lying and three-quarters-lying (see Figure 4.7c) are often chosen at first, but side-lying (see Figure 4.7b) is more supportive for the pelvis if the woman has any joint problems.

The recommended sequence for the relaxation is:

1. arms
2. legs
3. body
4. head
5. face
6. breathing

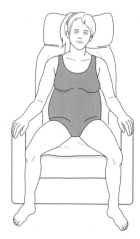

Figure 5.3   Position of ease.

Arms

Shoulders Pull your shoulders down towards your feet.
STOP pulling your shoulders down.
Feel that your shoulders are now lower and your neck feels longer.

Elbows Push your elbows slightly away from your side.
STOP pushing your elbows out.
Be aware that your elbows are open and slightly away from your side.

Hands Stretch out your hands, fingers and thumbs.
STOP stretching them out.
Observe that your hands, fingers and thumbs are fully supported.
Feel the surface on which they are resting.

Legs

Hips Roll your hips and knees outwards.
STOP rolling outwards.
Be aware that your legs are slightly apart and turned outwards.

Knees Adjust until comfortable.
STOP adjusting.
Reflect on the resulting position.

Feet Gently push your feet down, away from your face.
STOP pushing them down.
Feel your feet hanging loosely from the ankle joints.

Body

Press your body into the support.
STOP pressing.
Consider the sensation of your body resting against the support.

Head

Press your head into the pillow.
STOP pressing.
Feel your head nestling comfortably in the hollow you have made in the
pillow.

Face

Jaw Keeping your lips closed, pull down your lower jaw.
STOP pulling down.
Feel that your teeth are no longer touching and that the jaw-line is easy.

Tongue Move your tongue in your mouth.
STOP moving.
Register that your tongue is resting on the floor of your mouth.

Eyes Close your eyes, if you wish to, or stare instead.

Forehead Imagine someone smoothing away your frown lines from the
eye-brows up over the top of your head.
STOP doing this.
Feel the smoothing of the skin.

Breathing

Sigh out and breathe low down in your chest at your own natural
resting breathing rate, with slight emphasis on the out breath.

To prevent your brain being too active during your physical relaxation,
concentrate on something pleasant and happy which helps you to feel
comfortable. The whole sequence should be repeated probably a little
more quickly and then women and partners told how long they will be
left to relax.

This deep relaxation is often referred to as passive relaxation. At the end
of the period of relaxation, you should open your eyes and consider your
position – how open and unfolded you are compared with the position of
tension. Remember never to get up quickly following complete passive
relaxation. The circulation needs to be stimulated by stretching and performing foot and hand movements before sitting up slowly. After a minute
or two, full activity can be resumed. There is a very close link between

relaxation and breathing. It is very difficult to allow breathing to be calm and flow easily if one is tense, and difficult to relax if breathing is forced or controlled. Women and partners should be encouraged to increase their awareness by linking the two in practice and then using them as coping skills for labour (see Ch. 6) and everyday stresses. Women should be encouraged to practise the relaxation technique every day of their pregnancy, either sitting supported in an arm chair whilst watching television, or lying on the bed for an afternoon rest or in bed before going to sleep. Relaxation practised during pregnancy will help to lower blood pressure (Benson 1988). Fatigue and tension will be relieved and so there will be fewer aches and pains. The woman will be less anxious and the baby will gain too (Madders 1979).

Giving birth is, perhaps, the greatest athletic experience a woman is likely to take part in – both physically and emotionally. The woman may be fearful and anxious about the pain of labour, about her safety and that of her baby. For those delivering in the hospital, tension may be increased by the woman taking on a patient role. She may feel she will not have responsibility for her own labour and that she could lose control and dignity. In this respect, individuals vary enormously. To a lesser degree, the father may also have anxieties. The 'fight-flight' response will be made in response to pain, fear or apprehension and can lead to increased physical discomfort or pain and to inhibition of the uterine activity and dilatation of the cervix. With practice, relaxation can be used as a coping skill for labour (see Ch. 6). Energy is conserved and blood pressure kept lower by practising passive relaxation of voluntary muscles between contractions. During contractions, active relaxation can be used to raise the pain threshold, to increase the endurance to pain and allow labour to progress more easily. In order for the woman (and partner) to be able to use the relaxation skill actively for labour, frequent practice is essential. As well as using comfortable positions for training, it is necessary to try out this skill using postures that may be used in labour (see Ch. 6). Relaxation can be used postnatally, especially during disturbed nights or if the mother is anxious about coping with the new baby. It is also an aid to successful breastfeeding.

Before teaching relaxation, it is important for you to consider your attitude to this skill. Maybe you are only teaching it because you have to take your turn on the rota! Do you use it yourself? If not, should you begin to use it? Do you believe that it is an important coping technique for use in labour? Remember that your beliefs and views will filter through in your teaching however careful you try to be. You must have a full understanding of the method of relaxation you decide to teach, how it reduces tension and the value for the woman and partner during pregnancy, labour and the puerperium. Consider at what stage in your session you will include relaxation – it need not be left until the end. Think whether you will include it in each class. In order to use it effectively, women and partners need practice to learn the skill thoroughly. It is ideal to allow time in at least one session for this, but it is not cost-effective to spend one quarter of each session relaxing. It is a skill that should be practised every day at home to build up the woman's confidence for labour.

After learning the sequence and understanding the principles, it is necessary to try out the skill first on yourself. After that, it should be practised on one or two willing colleagues and friends who are not familiar with it. You will then need to consider how you intend to introduce relaxation to a group. Initially you could examine the causes and effects of stress with the women and their partners and exchange views on what stress-coping strategies they might use. This will also provoke discussion into the feelings of both partners. As a lead-in to teaching relaxation, the position of tension can be considered and actually felt by the group taking up a tense position and observing this on the other members of the group. The technique of choice should then be explained and the value of its use. Follow this by practice in a chosen position, repeating the sequence twice for the first few times. Progression is made during the weeks of practice by using less comfortable positions and a quicker, more active response in practice for labour along with breathing awareness. This will be the ripple relaxation where the sequence is run through quickly to gain a position of ease rapidly at the start of a contraction. At the end of the contraction, the ripple response is repeated.

The women (and partners) should always be told how long they will be relaxing if using the passive type. Usually, it will only be for a few minutes but refresher groups value this as time given to themselves and this baby and so enjoy longer relaxation. Background music can be used as an aid to relaxation and noise and interruption should be kept to a minimum (especially at first). However, as relaxation is for real life, the technique should gradually be used to switch off even from surrounding disturbance – after all, delivery suites are rarely totally quiet. Remember that the woman will need time to adjust before gradually moving from relaxation. She should be encouraged to stretch slowly and perform some movements of the feet and hands to stimulate the circulation before sitting and then standing.

Touch

Simple touch can be an excellent progression to use with couples or women working together in order to develop non-verbal communication based on touch (Kitzinger 1978). The partner learns to recognise areas of tension and the woman learns to respond to touch. Partners can place their hands gently but firmly on, for example, the shoulders in order to encourage low relaxation position. It offers women the chance to learn to relax while being touched, which will be practice for labour. Touching is also contact and a reminder to the woman that she is not alone.

Massage

For thousands of years, massage or laying on of hands has been used to heal and soothe. It is another means of contact, giving reassurance, warmth, pleasure, comfort and renewed vitality. Massage involves systematic stroking, effleurage, kneading and/or pressure of the soft tissues. It relieves pain by stimulating the natural production of endorphins and encephalins, and may also trigger the pain-gate closing mechanism (Wells 1994). The techniques can be introduced in antenatal sessions for benefit during pregnancy, labour and general living.

Aromatherapy

Aromatherapy is the use of essential oils, which can be administered in different ways. One drop of the chosen oil can be added to 5 mls of a carrier oil which can then be used as a massage medium for effleurage to any part of the body, but is especially relaxing on the back. Three or four drops can be added to warm bath water which should be swirled gently before the woman gets in to soak for 20–30 minutes. The oils can also be added to water and inhaled via a vaporizer warmed by a small candle. There are very many essential oils, which are available from chemists and health stores, but not all are suitable for pregnancy and some are contraindicated.

Imagery and suggestion

Imagery and suggestion may be incorporated into other relaxation techniques. Concentration is on a mental image rather than on the physical state. To give the mind something calm and pleasant to think about, many suggestions are given, for example, a walk under trees, a garden or a favourite scene. Music, carefully chosen, may be played in the background. Each woman and partner must choose for themselves what image is right for them, as some may cause tension rather than aid relaxation; for example, using waves of the sea may cause tension if someone is frightened of water.

Hypnosis

Hypnosis is described as an altered state of consciousness that is artificially induced and characterised by increased receptiveness to suggestions (Benson 1988). It is capable of producing an anaesthetic effect, but it is used infrequently in labour as it is very time-consuming and is not successful for everyone.

Transcendental meditation (TSM)

Transcendental meditation is a simple skill involving the use of a mantra – secret word, sound or phrase – by the woman. This is repeated over and over again whilst resting in a comfortable position and a quiet environment. Practice is required at least twice a day. TSM has been shown to produce the relaxation response. The woman would be deeply relaxed but mentally active (Benson, 1988).

Yoga

The technique of Yoga includes relaxation and breathing, and a woman who has used this method prior to pregnancy may choose to continue to practise it for childbirth. However as Yoga includes postures and stretching which may not be suitable for all pregnant women, the author advises women not to take up this technique for the first time when they become pregnant. Yoga teachers may, however, be trained in holding classes just for women in pregnancy which will be especially adapted to avoid exercises which could be harmful at this time. As with all exercise sessions women must be advised to check that the teachers are fully qualified.

Relaxation techniques are coping skills for life which, once really learnt, are never forgotten. Although educators aim at their use in labour and delivery, they should also encourage their application in everyday living to deal with stressful situations.

REFERENCES

Benson H 1988 The Relaxation Response. Collins, Glasgow
Holmes T H, Rahe R H 1967 The social readjustment rating scale. Journal of Psychosomatic Research 11:213
Jacobsen E 1938 Progressive Relaxation. University of Chicago Press, Chicago
Kitzinger S 1978 The Experience of Childbirth. 4th edn. Pelican Books, London
Madders J 1979 Stress and Relaxation. Martin Dunnitz, London
Mitchell L 1987 Simple Relaxation. 2nd edn. John Murray, London
Wells P E 1994 Manipulative procedures. In: Wells P E, Frampton V, Bowsher D (eds). Pain: Management in Physiotherapy. Butterworth Heinemann, Oxford
Woodrow Y 1988 Relaxation Techniques in Prenatal Education. In: Wilder E (ed) Obstetric and Gynecologic Physical Therapy. Churchill Livingstone, New York

FURTHER READING

Benson H 1998 The Relaxation Response. Collins, Glasgow
Madders J 1979 Stress and Relaxation. Martin Dunnitz, London
Mitchell L 1987 Simple Relaxation. John Murray, London

6

Coping strategies for labour

Problems in labour   69
Coping strategies   70
  Respiration in labour   70
  Comfortable positions for first stage
    labour   71
  S.O.S. breathing   72

End of first stage   73
Second stage of labour   74
Role of the partner in labour   77
Teaching coping strategies   78
  Rehearsal of labour   78
References   80

This chapter discusses the physical problems that arise in labour and describes coping strategies which may be practised by couples in antenatal classes. One of the main reasons couples give for attending antenatal preparation classes is that they want to learn about labour and how to cope. To prepare couples for labour, we need to look at the problems they may face and suggest some coping strategies that they might consider.

PROBLEMS IN LABOUR:

1. fear of the known or the unknown
2. pain of contractions
3. fear of being unable to cope
4. tension
5. hyperventilation.

The author has found that the first three are the most common problems volunteered by couples, the others being the possible consequences of the failure to deal adequately with these three.

As antenatal educators our aims should be to:

1. allay fear
2. discuss relief of pain
3. suggest coping strategies for use in labour
4. teach relaxation techniques
5. prevent hyperventilation.

Discussion, visual aids and visits to the delivery suite will all help to allay fear and to reassure the couples. A session devoted to the methods of pain relief available in the unit in which they will deliver will help them to make informed decisions when the time comes. Couples should be encouraged to discuss their care with their midwife and may wish to fill in a birth plan stating their preferences if all goes well – this is promoting choice (DOH 1993).

Sessions during which coping strategies are practised will help the woman through the contractions and build up her confidence so that she will be able to cope with each contraction as it comes. Weisenberg (1999) believed that having confidence in coping strategies can influence a woman's own pain-relieving agents and her immune response. If the woman is able to 'ride' her contractions, then tension and hyperventilation should be minimised or avoided.

COPING STRATEGIES

The teaching of coping skills for labour has changed throughout the years with emphasis today being on a psychophysical approach, which includes relaxation and breathing awareness and different positions. In the past, some suggested breathing techniques (psychoprophylaxis) interfered with the natural rhythm of respiration and sometimes led to hyperventilation and subsequent criticism of the teachers. The commonly accepted way of dealing with this nowadays is to allow the woman to recognise and respond to the needs of her own body. Teachers should revise their respiratory knowledge and the effects of various breathing techniques in labour.

Respiration in labour

Respiration is controlled automatically by the respiratory centre in the brain, which can be overridden by voluntary control. The respiratory centre responds to the level of carbon dioxide in the blood flowing through the centre. Any difference in this level of carbon dioxide will cause alterations in the rate or depth of respiration to normalise the level. Several factors cause the level to be altered, the commonest of which is exercise. Exercise uses energy and increases carbon dioxide output, which automatically causes the respiratory centre to alter the rate or depth of respiration until the level is normal once more. A typical example of this is the way our breathing alters involuntarily when we run up a flight of steps.

Other factors affecting the respiratory centre are fear, apprehension, excitement, anger, frustration and pain. Most of these are exhibited in labour together with strong uterine contractions, which use oxygen and produce excess carbon dioxide. If this occurs, the respiratory centre, which is more sensitive in pregnancy (Metcalfe et al 1988; Polden & Mantle 1990), will automatically correct the situation. However, if the woman voluntarily superimposes deep or rapid breathing, she is in danger of causing

ventilation or overbreathing. The symptoms of this state are very
asant and frightening – dizziness, pallor, sweating, palpitations and
ng in the face and/or extremities. Buxton (1965) found that hyper-
lation occurred frequently when levels of breathing were practised as
ychoprophylaxis. Women should be aware of the possibility and dangers of hyperventilation and how to correct the situation, should it arise,
by breathing into their own cupped hands to restore the carbon dioxide
level quickly. To avoid causing hyperventilation, antenatal teachers are
now discouraging the practice of deep or rapid breathing patterns in
labour and are instead, encouraging the mother to tune in to her own natural breathing rhythm and needs. This tuning in is often called breathing
awareness and is a calm, regular breathing which reinforces relaxation.

Of the two phases of respiration, expiration is the relaxing one. It is useful for women to concentrate on the outward breath and to practise tuning
into the slight pause before inspiration follows. We always breathe in
and no-one needs encouraging to do so, but on some occasions we need
reminding to breathe out, or to do so more slowly. Breathing should never
be a group activity where the members are instructed to breathe in and
breathe out in time with each other. Each person should be advised to
breathe at their own individual rate and to think especially about the outward breath. It is suggested that slow, deep breathing in labour gives better alveolar ventilation, which increases the oxygen intake and decreases
the carbon dioxide levels as necessary (Stradling 1984). This would be
more beneficial than the rapid shallow breathing formerly suggested. As
described in Chapter 5, relaxation and respiration are very closely linked
and to prevent hyperventilation in labour, practising the chosen relaxation
technique in a comfortable and appropriate position will promote natural
breathing awareness.

Comfortable positions for first stage labour

It is not known what causes the uterus to start contracting but it is documented that a more upright position, which keeps the baby's head in contact with the cervix, stimulates effective contractions (Roberts et al 1983). It
is also documented by Carbonne et al (1996) that a supine lying position
should be contraindicated as they found that oxygenation of the fetus was
decreased in this position compared to the left lateral position. So a more
upright position should be encouraged during the first stage of labour.

During the first stage, the labouring woman is trying to conserve her
energy and allow the dilatation of the cervix to take place without
attempting to resist the contractions. To achieve this, the couple will need
to acquire some coping skills to help them through this long, tedious and
often frustrating phase of labour. To facilitate relaxation in labour, the
technique should be tried out in comfortable positions during pregnancy.

Obviously no-one can predict what will be a comfortable position when labour is in progress, but the couple will have some alternatives to try. If the contractions are felt mainly in the back, the woman may find a forward leaning position comfortable. For instance, sitting astride a chair, kneeling with arms supported or standing leaning forward against a wall or partner, all relieve the weight from the lumbar spine. Many women are happier to be mobile during the first stage and some find relief with pelvic rocking and rhythmic pelvic gyrations during the contractions. Others may prefer to use a rocking chair, beanbag, armchair or birthing ball if available in the delivery suite. Some positions of ease are shown in Figure 6.1. The woman may need to change her position frequently depending on the distribution of pain and her choice of pain relief, and it has been shown that alteration of position during the first stage leads to productive uterine contractions (Gupta & Nikodem 2001). The physiological method of relaxation described in Chapter 5 is possible in any position. The shoulders and finger joints can be checked quickly at the start of the contraction (ripple effect). A general outline plan of action for a contraction may be helpful for the couple to practise. If the woman understands the importance of relaxing through the contraction, she is much more likely to do so. A positive approach to each one will help the relaxation, whereas a negative one will encourage tension. So a woman could be advised to:

1. greet the contraction positively
2. assume a comfortable position of ease
3. sigh out and check that her shoulders and hands are relaxed
4. tune in to her natural breathing rhythm throughout the contraction
5. give a sigh of relief at the end.

This 5-point approach forms a helpful coping routine for labour, which can be practised by the woman and her birthing partner antenatally. The woman will need to concentrate on coping with the contractions and may need to be reminded not to try to hold a conversation at the same time! It will be necessary for her to check her relaxation at the end of each contraction and, if there is time, to use the passive technique between contractions.

S.O.S. breathing

If, as labour progresses, the woman finds herself breathing more quickly and beginning to tense during the contractions, concentrating more on the outward breath and audibly sighing out the air may help. This Sighing Out Slowly breathing is often called **SOS** breathing and is used to prevent the emergency that could follow prolonged hyperventilation. Sighing out not only slows down the rate of breathing but also relaxes tense shoulders at the same time. The partner can breathe with her at her natural breathing rate.

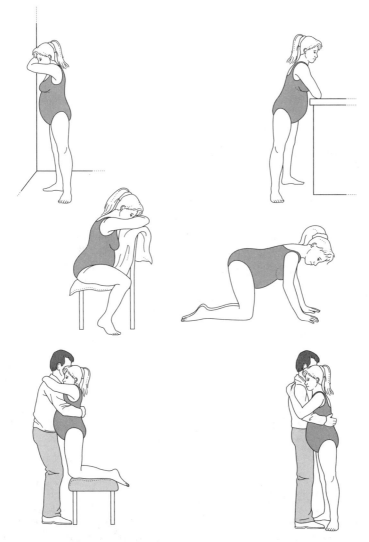

Figure 6.1 Alternative positions of ease for the first stage of labour.

End of first stage

It may be useful to adapt the breathing slightly towards the end of the first stage of labour if there is a premature desire to push. The instinctive reaction is to take in a deep breath, hold it and bear down unless advised not to do so. Alteration of position is the most effective way of avoiding premature pushing and the woman can be helped into a side-lying position or, more effective still, a kneeling position with head resting on

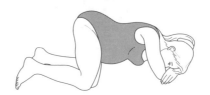

Figure 6.2   Knee-chest position to avoid pushing at the end of first stage.

forearms (see Figure 6.2). This will relieve the pressure from the anterior lip of the cervix.

However, interrupted breathing in threes will also help to prevent pushing. This breathing adaptation can be referred to as puff-puff-blow or pant-pant-blow breathing and its aim is to prevent the diaphragm from fixing and increasing intra-abdominal pressure. (Panting, as used briefly for the crowning of baby's head, could cause hyperventilation if used during these long contractions). By giving two short blow-breaths out followed by a longer outward breath, the diaphragm is not allowed to fix, so pushing and hyperventilation are avoided. This type of breathing also requires increased concentration and may therefore be a diversionary technique. Some women may actually prefer to say do-not-push or count one-two-three.

The woman will be emotionally and physically tired now and couples should be reminded of these aspects of the end of first stage, and partners warned that the mother-to-be may exhibit unusual behaviour and language at this time. This all helps to let off steam and aids relaxation but can be alarming for the labour companion if not prepared for it. The men can remind their partners that this emotional upset is very common at this time in labour and means that the second stage is about to commence.

Second stage of labour

Positions for the second stage of labour should be tried out in the antenatal classes. Squatting is an advantageous position for delivery as the pelvic outlet is 1 cm greater in the transverse diameter and 2 cm greater in the antero-posterior diameter resulting in an increase of 28% in area compared with the supine position (Russell, 1982). However not many women are able to squat comfortably, but need to discover this before deciding to give it a try in labour (see Figure 6.3).

Gardosi et al (1989) designed a birthing cushion which allowed supported squatting and showed that there were shorter second stages and fewer forceps deliveries in the group that used this position. They also reported that high kneeling, high sitting and standing postures also result in fewer forceps deliveries and less perineal trauma than a lying or

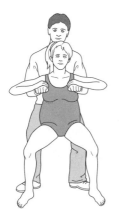
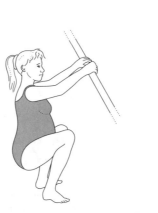
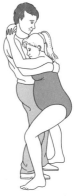

Figure 6.3 Squatting for second stage of labour.

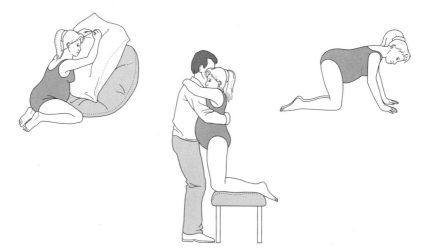

Figure 6.4 Kneeling for second stage of labour.

semi-recumbent position. An alternative which is often more acceptable is kneeling on all fours, leaning over a beanbag or the back of the bed or with arms round partner's neck (see Figure 6.4). Many women are comfortable in a high sitting position but should not be allowed to slip down into a lying posture or they will then be pushing uphill against gravity (see Figure 6.5). The abdominal muscles will not be able to work to their full potential if the woman is not curled forwards, as they will not be in their shortest position.

Gupta and Nikodem (2001) suggested several possible benefits of an upright posture (any upright or lateral position as against supine or

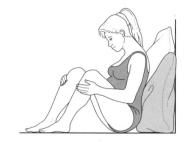

Figure 6.5 High sitting for second stage of labour.

lithotomy position) during second stage (see Box 6.1) and concluded that women should be encouraged to give birth in the position they find most comfortable.

Box 6.1 Benefits of an upright posture in second stage labour

- a slight reduction in length of second stage
- a small reduction in number of assisted deliveries
- a reduction in episiotomy rate
- less incidence of second degree perineal tears
- reduced reporting of severe pain in second stage
- fewer abnormal fetal heart rate patterns.

Distinct upright positions that are gravity assisted include:

1. high sitting
2. semi-recumbent
3. prone-kneeling
4. high kneeling
5. free squatting
6. squatting on birthing cushion.

The practice of resting the mother's feet on the midwife's hips has been discouraged for health and safety reasons in relation to the midwife. The extensor reflex pattern that this habit produced did not help the expulsive efforts and must have caused the midwife problems too.

Delivery positions for women with special needs may need to be discussed with a women's health physiotherapist. For example, a woman who has presented with diastasis symphysis pubis antenatally should keep abduction of the hips to a minimum. Kneeling or side lying may be the better positions for her delivery (Fry 1999). The issue of to push or not to push must rest with the individual midwife and mother-to-be.

The commonly taught method of pushing in the past was the use of the Valsalva manoeuvre, taking in a very deep breath, tucking the chin on the chest, closing the glottis and pushing for as long as possible. This was followed by a topping-up of breath and continued pushing for the duration of the contraction. The manoeuvre was so called after the physician of that name who used the procedure for expelling pus from the middle ear. In labour its use may lead to undesirable consequences, even loss of consciousness if maternal cerebral blood flow is already compromised (Bush, 1992). It must be borne in mind that prolonged breath-holding followed by prolonged pushing using the Valsalva manoeuvre may be harmful to a baby who is already compromised because holding the breath for more than 6 seconds decreases the fetal circulation (Caldeyro-Barcia 1979). This prolonged pushing also puts additional strain on the fascia of the linea alba, rectus sheath and pelvic floor (Noble 1995); a perineum which has had time to thin out gradually is less likely to require an episiotomy. It appears that it is better to discourage breath-holding and to encourage women to bear down as they would to empty their bowels when they have the urge to do so. Several such bearing-down actions may be needed during the contraction. On some occasions, the midwife may need to coach the labouring woman in pushing, particularly if the uterine contractions cannot be felt, for example, following top up of epidural anaesthetic.

Between the contractions, the woman will benefit from quick total relaxation, which will allow her circulation and breathing to revert to normal before she begins the hard work of the next contraction. She may need reminding to relax her pelvic floor when she is aware of the pressure of the baby' head on the perineum. This will minimise the discomfort caused by the gradual stretching. The ultimate stretch experienced at the actual crowning can be simulated in the antenatal class to some extent by placing the little fingers in the corners of the mouth and pulling the lips sideways. The splitting/burning sensation is slightly similar to that felt in all diameters by those women who have not been given an episiotomy. The mouth seems to be empathetic with the pelvic floor and it is suggested that if the mouth is slack then the pelvic floor will also be relaxed (Kitzinger 1977). Deep panting or blowing out will prevent pushing at the crowning and, at this stage, is unlikely to cause ventilatory problems. The woman may need to be reminded to work with her midwife at this time and her partner can help by reinforcing instructions.

ROLE OF THE PARTNER IN LABOUR

Partners can play a very important role in the birth of their baby but only if both parents-to-be wish it. Men should not be forced into a position where they are not totally happy because they feel it is expected of them. Neither should the woman feel that she must have a companion if she would rather not. She might prefer to have a friend or female relative with her, but usually women in a stable relationship choose their partner (who may be female). Apart from being a companion and an emotional and physical support, the partner can be responsible for various tasks, which will not only help the woman but will also assist the staff. For ease, in the following section the birthing partner will be referred to as 'he'.

Ideally the couple will have attended at least one joint session on labour, better still a whole course, so the birthing partner can reinforce coping mechanisms learnt at the classes, particularly breathing and relaxation techniques. He may even breathe in time with her during the contractions and he is ideally placed to recognise if his partner starts to tense or panic-breathe. He can reinforce instructions from the midwifery staff and remind his partner of the milestones reached along the way. It is very comforting for the woman to have a close companion with whom she can completely relax and share her doubts and worries and enjoy the physical reassurance that close contact can bring. This contact may take the form of merely holding hands, stroking, brow-mopping or massage. The partner can be the one to help the woman into different positions as labour progresses and to support her in her chosen position during the second stage contractions. Between the contractions, he may find himself stretching or massaging her legs and feet as cramp is a common problem at this time. Finally, his presence and active support at the actual birth is the start of a new family life that both partners will share.

TEACHING COPING STRATEGIES

Teaching relaxation has been discussed in Chapter 5, but it might be helpful to hold a rehearsal of labour for couples and talk through imaginary contractions whilst they adopt any of the different positions that have been suggested.

Rehearsal of labour

The following is just an example of how the labour strategies might be introduced to a class.

Early first stage

"You may feel the very early contractions as slight backache or period pains but they are more uncomfortable than painful. They may last up to 40 seconds and may be up to 30 minutes apart. If it is night-time try to rest, but during the day you may prefer to carry on with everyday activities, have a light snack, relax in a warm bath or pass the time watching television."

First stage contractions

"The contractions are now stronger and you may describe them as very uncomfortable or even painful. They may last 50 to 60 seconds and be 5 to 10 minutes apart. You may wish to remain active but concentrate on each contraction as it comes. Now is the time to put your 5-point plan into action:

1. greet the contraction positively and sigh out
2. check that you are in a comfortable position
3. check shoulders and hands are relaxed
4. breathe low down in your chest and concentrate on the outward breath. As the contraction rises to a peak, continue to breathe easily throughout
5. give a sigh of relief at the end as the contraction dies away, and check you are relaxed."

Later first stage contractions

"By now the contractions will be very strong, may last about 60 seconds and be only 2 to 3 minutes apart. You may have had some form of pain relief and prefer to be less active. The contraction will be at its peak for about 45 seconds and you will feel as though it is taking over your whole body – let it, don't try to resist or fight it. Your 5-point plan still holds good but you may need to concentrate on Sighing Out Slowly during the contraction – your partner can do it with you. Stay relaxed and don't forget the long sigh at the end."

End of first stage (transition)

"This is a transitional stage before the uterus starts to push the baby down the birth canal. The contractions now are very powerful and long and may be every 2 minutes. You may feel or be sick and there may be pressure on your back passage, which makes you want to push at the peak of the contraction. Never push until your midwife has confirmed that you are in the second stage – instead roll onto your side or into the kneeling position with your head on your forearms. This is where the breathing-in-threes technique should help you through the contraction. At the end of this one you deserve two sighs of relief!

You have been working very hard and will feel emotionally and physically drained. You may think that you cannot carry on any longer, you may even turn on your partner and tell him to go. These are recognisable reactions at this time and mean that there is not much longer to go before you are in the second stage".

Second stage contractions

"Sometimes the contractions diminish for a short time after full dilatation of the cervix. You can make the most of this short rest by relaxing. When the contractions return you will probably feel as though you want to bear down with them, but there is no need to push unless you have the urge to do so. When you are pushing, adopt your chosen position and bear down steadily, remembering not to hold your breath. You may need four or five bearing down pushes with each contraction. Relax completely between contractions and breathe slowly and deeply. Gradually you will feel the pressure of your baby's head stretching your perineum; this is when you need to relax your pelvic floor during the contractions."

Crowning

"As the baby's head is stretching the perineum to its limit, you will feel a tight, burning sensation. Stay calm and listen to your midwife. She will tell you to stop pushing and to pant deeply just for a few seconds, then to push, perhaps to pant again and then push again. This will allow your baby's head to be born slowly. During the next contraction you may be asked to pant again as the shoulders are delivered, the rest of the baby will slide out easily. At last the hard work is over – Congratulations!"

REFERENCES

Bush A 1992 Cardiopulmonary effects of pregnancy and labour. Journal of the Association of Chartered Physiotherapists in Obstetrics and Gynaecology 71:3–4

Buxton R St J 1965 Breathing in labour: the influence of psychoprophylaxis. Nursing Mirror 1965;viii

Caldeyro-Barcia R 1979 The influence of maternal bearing-down efforts during second stage on fetal well-being. Birth and Family Journal 6:7–22

Carbonne B, Benachi A, Leveque M L et al 1996 Maternal position during labor: effects on fetal oxygen saturation measured by pulse oximetry. Obstetrics and Gynecology 88(5):797–800

Department of Health (DOH) 1993 Changing Childbirth: report of the expert maternity group. HMSO London 1993

Fry D 1999 Perinatal symphysis pubis dysfunction; a review of the literature. Journal of the Association of Chartered Physiotherapists in Women's Health 85:11–18

Gardosi J, Sylvester S, B-Lynch C 1989 Alternative positions in the second stage of labour: a randomised controlled trial. British Journal of Obstetrics and Gynaecology 96(11):1290–1296

Gupta J K, Nikodem V C 2001 Woman's position during second stage of labour (Cochrane Review). In: The Cochrane Library Issue 4, Oxford: Update Software

Kitzinger S 1977 Education and Counselling for Childbirth. Baillière Tindall, London

Metcalfe J, Stocks M K, Barron D H 1988 Maternal physiology during gestation. In: Knobil E, Neill J (eds) The Physiology of Reproduction. Raven Press, New York

Noble E 1995 Essential Exercises for the Childbearing Year. New Life Images, Harwich USA

Polden M, Mantle J 1990 Physiotherapy in Obstetrics and Gynaecology. Butterworth Heinemann, London

Roberts J E, Mendez-Bauer C, Wodell D A 1983 The effects of maternal position on uterine contractility and efficiency. Birth 10:243–249

Russell J G B 1982 The rationale of primitive delivery positions. British Journal of Obstetrics and Gynaecology 89:712–715

Stradling J 1984 Respiratory physiology during labour. Midwife, Health Visitor and Community Nurse 20:38–42

Weisenberg M 1999 Cognitive aspects of pain In: Wall P D, Melzack R (eds) Textbook of Pain. Churchill Livingstone, Edinburgh

7

Transcutaneous electrical nerve stimulation (TENS)

Advantages of TENS in
    labour   84
Electrodes   85
    Siting the electrodes   85
TENS hire   87

Criteria for selection of a TENS
    unit   87
TENS for post-caesarean delivery   88
References   89
Further reading   90

This chapter introduces the concepts of transcutaneous electrical nerve stimulation (TENS). It describes the advantages of TENS and its use during labour and discusses the criteria relevant when selecting a particular unit.

Transcutaneous electrical nerve stimulation (TENS or TNS) has been used as a method of pain relief for many years and is widely used today, particularly for chronic pain and pain associated with terminal illness. More recently it has been used for more acute pain and found to be of advantage (Woolf 1999). In 1983 Spembly manufactured a TENS unit especially designed for use in labour. This was the first unit of its type in the UK and is called the Obstetric Pulsar (see Figure 7.1). Since then, other manufacturers have adapted existing models with varying degrees of success. Criteria for selection of an effective unit appear later in the chapter.

TENS is a low-frequency current applied to the skin via pairs of electrodes. These can be placed over the painful area or over the nerve routes supplying the area of pain. The current produces a tingling sensation, the intensity (strength) of which can be altered by the individual. The pulsed low-frequency modality encourages the release of cerebrospinal endogenous opiates (endorphins and encephalins) which are the body's own natural pain-relieving agents and these raise the individual's pain threshold (Thompson 1989). The obstetric model differs in that it has a high-frequency modality which, when activated, brings in a continuous high-frequency current to boost the low-frequency current to give added pain relief. It is thought that this higher frequency current works on the pain-gate theory and lessens the pain impulses received by the brain (Wall, 1985). The high-frequency modality is brought into play by pressing a patient-demand switch and stopped by pressing it once more.

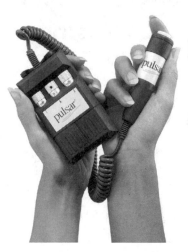

Figure 7.1 A Tens unit (Courtesy of Spembly Medical Limited).

ADVANTAGES OF TENS IN LABOUR (see Box 7.1)

There are no side effects from TENS and no depression of respiration (Woolf 1999) – a pacemaker in situ being the only contraindication to its use. It is a safe, non-invasive therapy which, if required, can be used in conjunction with other forms of pain relief as labour progresses. TENS does not give a pain-free labour and this fact must be stressed to the woman and her partner. However, for the woman who wishes to be in control of her pain relief it is a useful addition to other available analgesia. The general feeling among midwives is that TENS users who choose to have additional analgesia require lower doses than those who are not using TENS. This is supported by Kaplan et al (1998) who described TENS as being

---

Box 7.1 Advantages of TENS in labour

- self-regulated/self-administered
- releases the body's own pain-relieving agents
- non-invasive, drug-free
- no drowsiness – user remains alert and co-operative
- no known side effects
- allows freedom of movement and any position
- does not alter the course of labour
- can be stopped at any time
- can be used in conjunction with other forms of pain relief.

an effective non-pharmacological and non-invasive adjuvant pain relief modality for use in labour and delivery. They claimed that not only did the use of TENS reduce the amount of analgesic drugs, but also slightly reduced the duration of the first stage of labour. However Carroll et al (1997) claimed that randomised controlled trials provided no compelling evidence for TENS having an analgesic effect during labour. TENS can be used during suturing and to relieve afterpains as well as during labour itself.

TENS works best for women who apply it early in labour as it takes about 40 minutes for the endorphins to be maximally released (Salar et al 1981). It can help the woman to cope in the early latent phase before labour is fully established. It has been shown that the levels of pain and distress-related thoughts experienced during the latent phase of labour were predictive of the length of labour and obstetric outcomes (Wuitchik et al 1989). If a woman is going to have labour induced, it is suggested that she activates the TENS unit on the low-frequency mode 30–40 minutes before the procedure is commenced. When she feels in need of further pain relief, she can activate the high-frequency mode at the start of the contraction and use for the duration of the contraction, returning to the low-frequency mode at the end.

ELECTRODES

For labour, four electrodes, which are of sufficient length to cover the nerve roots supplying the uterus and cervix (T10 – L1) and the birth canal and pelvic floor (S2 – S4), are required. The recommended size of the electrodes is 10 cm × 4 cm, and they can be of different materials. The original and most economical electrodes are made of carbon-impregnated rubber, which needs a coupling medium of gel under the complete surface to ensure continuous contact with the skin. More recently, disposable electrodes have been introduced which are applied to a wet skin and are self-adherent. A third type (supplied with hire units) has a very sticky self-adhesive surface and in theory can be re-used a few times, but in practice this is not recommended for reasons of hygiene and because the electrodes become less adhesive.

Siting the electrodes

The woman should sit on the edge of the bed whilst her partner stands behind on the other side of the bed. She should have her arms relaxed by her side and her back exposed down to the gluteal cleft. The area from the level of the bra strap down to the gluteal cleft should be washed and dried to remove any natural skin grease that could impede the electrical current. The electrodes are attached to the leads making sure no metal is exposed. To site the upper two electrodes, the T10 vertebra is palpated. The easiest way of locating this is to feel for the inferior angle of the scapula with the little fingers of each hand, then reach across to the spine at the same level with the thumbs. The vertebra palpated by the thumbs will be T7, count three vertebrae down to find T10. (A good guide is the lower border of the bra clips in most women). The upper borders of one set of electrodes should be fixed at the level of T10 about 2 cm either side of the thoracic spine (approx 5 cm apart), with the leads hanging downwards (see Figure 7.2). If the re-usable carbon electrodes are being used, they should be thoroughly covered with the conducting gel supplied and held in place with a piece of Mefix, large enough to cover both electrodes. The top of the second pair of electrodes is placed at the level of the sacral dimples (S2) with the lower borders reaching down to just above the gluteal cleft. The leads should point upwards (see Figure 7.2).

The electrodes should not be placed on the abdomen as there may be a slight chance of interference on the fetal monitor if a scalp electrode is in use. It has been reported that interference has been noted occasionally when both sets of electrodes are placed dorsally, but this has been with older monitors and disappears when the intensity of the TENS is reduced. With both sets of electrodes in place and checked and the unit switched off, the plug end of each lead is inserted into the sockets on the top of the TENS unit. The woman should know which electrodes are attached to which control so she can increase the intensity of each channel independently. A much better effect is achieved if the woman is in complete control of the unit from the start. Once the electrodes are in place, the TENS unit can be clipped on to her clothes and she can remain active or adopt any position she wishes.

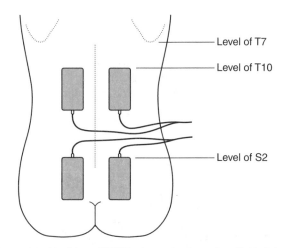

Level of T7

Level of T10

Level of S2

Figure 7.2 Position of TENS electrodes for pain relief in labour.

The intensity (strength) of the two channels can be increased as required using the relevant intensity control (see Figure 7.1). The frequency of the pulses, which is a personal choice, can also be varied by altering the rate control (see Figure 7.1). This does not affect the intensity of the output, only the rate of the pulses. The manufacturers of the Spembly Pulsar unit advise an initial frequency of 7 on the dial, then further adjustment to meet the personal needs of each individual. However, some TENS units have a pre-set unalterable frequency.

Ideally women and their partners should be introduced to the TENS unit during the antenatal classes. Then if they are interested in trying or applying it, a group or individual session can be arranged where the women can experience its sensation on their backs and their partners practise siting the electrodes (see Ch. 10). The sensation on the back is usually preferred to that on the forearm and women like to feel it before going to the expense of hiring a unit.

TENS HIRE

Unless a delivery suite has sufficient units to allow women to take one home just prior to their expected delivery date, hiring their own is often preferred. The hired units will include the easy-to-apply, self-adhesive electrodes which do not require gel. There will be two pairs for use in labour and generally, depending on the company, an additional pair for practice in the two weeks prior to birth. Various companies supply units for hire and costs depend on the package offered. Hire contracts vary between four and six weeks with nearly all companies offering a free extension period as long as they are notified in advance. The more expensive hire charges include a demonstration video, spare batteries and pre-paid return packaging (see Figure 7.3). Obstetric TENS units are for use in labour only and should not be used for anything else. Their use is contraindicated before 37 weeks of pregnancy because of the slight risk of preterm labour. Some delivery suites hire out their own units, but this can be an onerous undertaking. A new battery and electrodes are needed for each user and the unit should be checked after its return to the labour suite before being re-issued.

CRITERIA FOR SELECTION OF A TENS UNIT

Midwives and health visitors should be aware of the different models on the market before giving out literature to couples. The cheapest deal is not necessarily the best option. Crothers (1992) tried out two different units during her own labour and decided that certain criteria were important. She was a member of the working party of The Association of Chartered

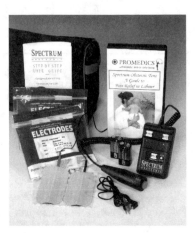

Figure 7.3 A TENS hire package (Courtesy of Promedics Limited, UK).

Physiotherapists in Obstetrics and Gynaecology (now Women's Health) who devised the following criteria for the suitability of TENS equipment for use in labour:

- sufficient intensity/amplitude to relieve pain
- scope to alter the frequency
- both pulsed and continuous mode
- additional amplitude with continuous mode
- simple and easy to apply and operate
- correct instructions for placing the electrodes
- press/release booster button, not press/hold
- electrodes to measure a minimum of 10 cm × 4 cm
- separate intensity control for each pair of electrodes
- durable electrodes, leads and attachments
- transmission gel must be suitable for adequate conduction with carbon electrodes.

All units should conform to safety standard BS 5724.

TENS FOR POST-CAESAREAN DELIVERY

Following caesarean section, where the mother is not offered self-administered pain relief via Cardiff pump or an epidural, TENS may be used for post-operative pain relief. It has been found that women who used TENS after caesarean births required less narcotic analgesia and so were better able to cope with their babies (Hollinger 1986). The electrodes are usually placed above a Pfannenstiel incision towards the outer sides of the abdomen as this is where most pain is felt (see Figure 7.4).

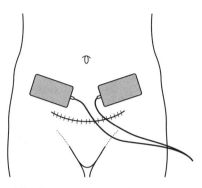

Figure 7.4 Position of TENS electrodes for relief of post-caesarean wound pain.

One set of electrodes only may be applied, or a second pair may be placed either side of the first and second lumbar vertebrae. The low-frequency mode is all that is necessary at rest, but, if the mother needs to cough or move about, the high-frequency can be used as during contractions.

The UKCC's advice with regard to midwives using TENS is contained in the following Registrar's Letter 8/1991:

"The Council has accepted the recommendation of its Midwifery Committee that midwives may, on their own responsibility, manage pain relief in labour by the use of transcutaneous nerve stimulation (TNS) provided that:

1. they have received adequate and appropriate *instruction*, which is a matter to be determined by agreed local policy and
2. *safety standards* conform to those laid down by the Department of Health Medical Devices Directorate in England, or equivalent body in Scotland, Wales or Northern Ireland. The current standard for all medical equipment is set out in British Standard specification BS 5724 Part 1 1989".

REFERENCES

Carroll D, Tramer M, McQuay H et al 1997 Transcutaneous electrical nerve stimulation in labour pain: a systematic review. British Journal of Obstetrics and Gynaecology (2):169–175
Crothers E 1992 TENS in labour. Journal of the Association of Chartered Physiotherapists in Obstetrics and Gynaecology 70:26
Hollinger J L 1986 Transcutaneous electric nerve stimulation after caesarean birth. Physical Therapy 66:36
Kaplan B, Rabinerson D, Lirie S et al 1998 Transcutaneous electric nerve stimulation (TENS) for adjuvant pain-relief during labour and delivery. International Journal of Gynaecology and Obstetrics 60(3):251–255
Salar G, Job I, Mingrino S et al 1981 Effect of transcutaneous electrotherapy on CSF beta endorphin content in patients without pain problems. Pain 10:169–172

Thompson J W 1989 Pharmacology of Transcutaneous Electrical Nerve Stimulation (TENS). Journal of the Intractable Pain Society of Great Britain and Ireland 7:33–40

Wall P D 1985 The discovery of transcutaneous electrical nerve stimulation. Physiotherapy 71:348–350

Woolf C J 1999 Transcutaneous and implanted nerve stimulation. In: Wall P D, Melzack R (eds) Textbook of Pain. Churchill Livingstone, Edinburgh

Wuitchik M, Bakal D, Lipshitz J 1989 The clinical significance of pain and cognitive activity in latent labour. Obstetrics and Gynecology 73:35–42

FURTHER READING

Wall P D, Melzack R (eds) 1999 Textbook of Pain. Churchill Livingstone, Edinburgh

Physiological changes and physical problems in the puerperium

Physiological changes 91
  Cardiovascular 92
  Musculoskeletal 92
Some physical postnatal
  problems 93
  A bruised and
    oedematous
    perineum 93
  Haematoma 94
  Haemorrhoids 94

Diastasis recti 94
Symphysis pubis dysfunction
  (SPD) 95
Backache 95
Coccydynia 95
Urinary problems 96
Bowel problems 97
Dyspareunia 97
Fatigue 97
References 98

This chapter describes the changes occurring in the postpartum period and some of the physical problems women may encounter.

PHYSIOLOGICAL CHANGES

Most of the physiological changes which occurred due to the hormonal influences during pregnancy (see Ch. 2) gradually resolve during the six to eight weeks following delivery, so that at the end of the puerperium the mother should be back to her pre-pregnancy state. Some systems revert more quickly than others. The musculoskeletal system can still manifest some effects as long as six months postpartum (Polden & Mantle 1990) which has a bearing on the exercises and advice that should be given to women at this time.

The main physiological changes that occur during the puerperium are:

- involution of the uterus which starts immediately following delivery and should be complete after six weeks
- lactation which occurs as a result of the action of prolactin initially secreted by the anterior pituitary gland
- physiological changes in other body systems which return the body to its pre-pregnancy state.

The important ones to note here, because of their effect on the physical rehabilitation of the postnatal mother are the cardiovascular and musculoskeletal changes.

Cardiovascular

Smooth muscle tone in the walls of the veins begins to improve, blood volume decreases, the viscosity of the blood returns to normal and cardiac output and blood pressure drop to their pre-pregnant levels. There may be some residual oedema in the feet and hands from pregnancy, from increased fluid input in labour, from congestion due to prolonged pushing in the second stage or from relative immobility immediately postpartum. There is a slightly increased risk of deep vein thrombosis and possible embolus.

Musculoskeletal

The levels of relaxin and progesterone (see Ch. 2) reduce to normal within seven days postpartum but their effects on the fibrous tissue, muscles and ligaments may take four to five months to be reversed (Calguneri et al 1982). It has been suggested that it can take up to six months before joint laxity regresses to near its pre-pregnancy state (Polden & Mantle 1990), and Horsley (1998) reported clinicians finding postural changes and muscle weakness up to 12 months postpartum. In the immediate postpartum period, the ligaments are at their longest and the joints are at their least stable meaning that the mother is at her most vulnerable for musculoskeletal problems.

The abdominal muscles are stretched and weakened. The length of the abdominals increases by approximately 115% (Gilleard & Brown 1996). There could also be diastasis of the rectus abdominis muscles due to the hormonal effect on the linea alba coupled with the increasing bulk of the uterus. Persistent use of the Valsalva manoeuvre during the second stage of labour (see Ch. 6) increases the stress on the abdominal muscles and may be a contributory factor to diastasis (Noble 1995).

The pelvic floor muscles have supported the weight of the uterus and contents during pregnancy and have been stretched during delivery. It is documented that pregnancy, regardless of the mode of delivery, greatly increases the prevalence of pelvic floor dysfunction (MacLennan et al 2000). The composition of the fascial layer of the pelvic floor has altered due to the hormonal influence of relaxin and has been strained by the increased weight of the pelvic contents during pregnancy (see Ch. 2). It too will have stretched at delivery and will take time to resume its pre-pregnant form. The perineum may have been torn or cut and repaired and may be bruised, swollen and sore. It is possible that there could be some degree of urinary incontinence in the early puerperium. It has been suggested that some women lose control over their pelvic floor muscles following intense postpartum perineal pain (Shepherd, 1980).

SOME PHYSICAL POSTNATAL PROBLEMS

A bruised and oedematous perineum

This can be extremely painful and incapacitating for the new mother. Advice about positions for feeding may help the mother's comfort; sitting with a pillow under each ischial tuberosity to relieve the pressure on the perineum or side-lying with a pillow between the knees. Some units may have specially constructed inflatable cushions, which are helpful in taking weight off the perineum. These cushions can be inflated to suit individual comfort and appear to have all the advantages of a rubber ring without the disadvantages. A very comfortable resting position is prone-lying with a pillow under the hips and another under the head and shoulders. This takes the pressure off the perineum but the mother may need more pillows if her breasts are tender. Many new mothers forget that they can lie on their tummies once more!

A painful perineum can be eased considerably by the application of cold therapy, which has many benefits for recent injuries (see Box 8.1). Cold therapy may be administered in the form of flaked or crushed ice, which is cheap, readily available and easy to apply. It may be placed inside a polythene bag or gauze that is covered with a clean disposable towel and placed on the painful area for 10–15 minutes. If the mother is applying ice to her own perineum she should be reminded of the risks of a burn if the ice remains in contact with the skin. However, the painful area can be massaged for 5–10 minutes by an ice cube held in a disposable cloth. Ice should not be used for longer than the advised length of time and should be crushed if in continuous contact to avoid the possibility of ice burns.

Box 8.1 Benefits of cold therapy for recent injuries

- reduction in bleeding
- reduction in swelling
- alleviation of pain
- release of local endorphins
- reduction of muscle spasm

The pain-relieving properties of ice for recent injuries have been consistently documented (Low & Reed 2000, Palastanga 1994). Moore and James (1989) compared the application of Epifoam, hamamelis water and ice. Each gave good pain relief to two thirds of the women on the first day, but ice gave better pain relief on subsequent days. The most comfortable position for the mother is usually side-lying on an inco-pad, with a pillow between her knees. Much discussion has taken place about the use of ice delaying healing (Grant et al 1989) but Low & Reed (2000) and Palastanga (1994) stated that the initial vasoconstriction which is followed by a vasodilatation will increase circulation and promote healing and Steen & Cooper (1998) found there was no clear evidence to suggest that cold therapy would result in delayed wound healing. An alternative to ice is the gel pack, which is now readily available and easy to apply. Steen et al (2000) evaluated the effectiveness of a maternity gel pack compared with ice packs and epifoam in relieving perineal trauma and found that not only were the gel packs more effective but that the women rated them more highly.

A women's health physiotherapist will be able to treat the perineum with therapeutic ultrasound or pulsed electromagnetic energy (PEME). The latter is sometimes called pulsed shortwave, although this term is not technically correct, and is very often referred to as *Megapulse* or *Curapulse* which are actually the trade names for particular models. Both ultrasound and PEME have similar physiological effects, relieving pain and reducing oedema, but there is no evidence that the rate of healing is speeded up by treatment with either modality (Grant et al 1989). In a review of the literature to determine whether therapeutic ultrasound is a safe and effective treatment for acute perineal pain, persistent perineal pain and/or dyspareunia following childbirth, Hay-Smith (2002) concluded there was insufficient evidence to make a conclusion about the benefits or otherwise of therapeutic ultrasound for the above problem. Pelvic floor exercises in themselves help to relieve the pressure on the perineum especially in standing or sitting. The rhythmical contraction and relaxation of the muscles helps to improve the local circulation and remove waste products from the area.

Haematoma

Haematomata may occur in the perineum after vaginal delivery, particularly after instrumental delivery, or in the rectus sheath after caesarean delivery. Haematomata respond very favourably to the application of ultrasound or PEME administered by the women's health physiotherapist.

Haemorrhoids

Haemorrhoids are common after childbirth and may persist in up to 25% of women (Brown & Lumley 1998). Immediately postpartum they may be helped by the application of ultrasound or PEME. The haemorrhoids are visibly reduced in size in a short space of time and the accompanying pain alleviated.

Diastasis recti (see Ch. 3)

This is a condition where a gap of 2.5 cm (two fingers) or more appears between the two rectus muscles (Noble 1995). It can occur towards the end of pregnancy when it is difficult to detect, or may occur during labour but it is postnatally that the condition is most obvious. It is more common with multiple pregnancies, large babies and polyhydramnios, but may appear for seemingly no apparent reason in slim, fit women. It is thought that this might be due to altered collagen make-up. In severe cases, where the gap may be as much as 10 cms or more, the mother may complain of constant backache as the abdominal muscles are no longer supporting the spine or pelvis. It can be a frightening condition for a mother as the intestines may be visible and she may feel that they may protrude even further on standing. It is easy to detect a severe diastasis from the visible 'doming' of the recti on attempting to sit up from the supine position, but each mother should be examined individually. Testing for diastasis recti is described in Chapter 9 and treatment/advice is covered in detail in Chapter 3.

Symphysis pubis dysfunction (SPD) (see Ch. 3)

This condition, which was formerly known as diastasis symphysis pubis, may present in late pregnancy due to hormonal influence or may occur as a result of the trauma of a difficult labour (Fry 1999). Occasionally, however, the onset of symptoms can appear 24–48 hours after delivery and is thought to be caused by swelling and increased pressure within the confines of the joint (Driessen 1987). SPD appears to be underdiagnosed (McIntosh 1993; Scriven et al 1995) but has been more widely reported in recent times. (Assessment and treatment are covered in Ch. 3.)

Backache

In the early postnatal period, backache is usually postural, unless the woman was troubled with joint or ligament problems during her pregnancy. If she chose epidural anaesthesia for labour, the woman may have adopted a poor back position without realising it. Advice on posture and positions, how to get in and out of bed and lifting are all necessary (see Figures 4.8, 9.7). Pelvic tilting/rocking exercises should ease the backache. Local heat from a warm bath, heat lamp (or hot water bottle wrapped in towels if at home) may give comfort. Very weak abdominals or a significant diastasis of recti will lead to an alteration in posture and low back pain (Boissonnault and Kotarinos 1988). It is thought that there could be a connection between long-term backache and epidural anaesthesia in labour (see Ch. 3).

Coccydynia

Coccydynia may be related to a previous injury, but is more usually caused by a difficult delivery. The pain may result from a bruised or displaced coccyx or rarely from a fracture (Brunskill & Swain 1987). It is a very painful condition, which can incapacitate the mother, and alternative positions for feeding etc. must be suggested. Many mothers find prone-lying on a pillow is a comfortable resting position. If the mother wants to sit, pillows can be arranged so there is no pressure on the coccyx, and an upright position will be the most comfortable. An inflatable cushion can be adjusted to give minimal pressure on the area and can be hired for use at home. Pain relief will almost definitely be required. A women's health physiotherapist can apply ultrasound or PEME (see p96) or interferential therapy for pain relief. This latter is a further electrotherapy modality that can be successful in relieving pain. It has been suggested that gentle mobilisations may also be helpful, and that TENS can be a valuable means of analgesia (Polden & Mantle 1990).

Urinary problems (see Ch. 3)

Following delivery there is a physiological diuresis due to reduction in blood volume and increase in waste products. Some mothers, especially after an instrumental delivery, find it difficult to initiate micturition. They may be helped by performing regular pelvic-floor contractions in a warm bath. Alternatively, the mother may find that she is having difficulty in holding her urine long enough to get to the toilet and again pelvic-floor exercises should help these early problems.

Many women find that they leak a little urine when they cough, laugh, sneeze, lift objects or perform sudden movements. This symptom, known as stress incontinence, is common in pregnancy due to the hormonal influence on the pelvic floor plus the extra weight it is supporting (see Ch. 2). However it is generally thought that as many as one in three of all women who have had children suffer from this condition to a greater or lesser degree postnatally (Wilson et al 1996; Mørkved & Bø 1999), and Marshall et al (1996) claimed that as many as 59% of Irish women surveyed post-partum admitted symptoms of incontinence. In a study in 1990, it was found that 80% of primiparous women who had undergone vaginal deliveries showed electromyographic evidence of re-innervation of the pelvic-floor muscles eight weeks postpartum (Allen et al 1990), showing that some denervation had taken place at delivery.

Most cases of stress incontinence will respond to an individually-designed course of pelvic-floor exercises and all mothers who have symptoms which persist after 12 weeks must be encouraged to get a referral to a women's health physiotherapist either through their general practitioner or consultant, as women must be assessed and properly instructed in the performance of pelvic floor exercises (Bump et al 1991).

Other common problems which may manifest themselves postnatally are frequency, urgency and prolapse. Following assessment, these conditions can respond favourably to an individual regime of bladder training, pelvic-floor exercises and electrotherapy and so should be referred to a women's health physiotherapist (see Ch. 3).

Bowel problems

Fortunately faecal incontinence is much less common than urinary incontinence postnatally, but when present is an extremely distressing and embarrassing problem. It may be due to tearing or stretching of the anal sphincter or actual damage to the nerve supply to the pelvic-floor muscles (Snooks et al 1985). Swash (1993) stated that childbirth is responsible for most cases of faecal incontinence in women and MacArthur et al (2001) found that women delivered by forceps had almost twice the risk of developing faecal incontinence. Depending on the severity of the nerve damage, function may not be restored for some weeks or in some cases it may be permanently impaired. Sultan et al (1993) found that anal sphincter damage was more likely in primiparous women and that 35% of the women they followed up still suffered from faecal incontinence 16 months after childbirth. All women complaining of faecal incontinence should be referred for specialist help from a women's health physiotherapist.

Constipation is a problem for many women postnatally and may be avoided by advice on diet, exercise and correct defaecation techniques.

Dyspareunia

Dyspareunia (painful intercourse) can be a most distressing side effect of labour. It is more common in women who have had episiotomies (Kitzinger & Walters 1981) and three times more common in women who have had instrumental deliveries (Glazener et al 1997). It may resolve over the following few weeks or last much longer. It has been stated that 23% of women report pain during intercourse as long as three months after delivery (Sleep et al 1984). If after trying alternative positions and the use of lubricants, the condition persists, the woman should be referred for physiotherapy treatment. McIntosh (1988) found that of 22 women who complained of dyspareunia at three months postpartum, only five did not experience any relief of symptoms after 12 treatments of ultrasound. Hay-Smith (2002) did not find any conclusive evidence for the use of ultrasound, but it has been suggested that some relief may be gained from the counselling and reassurance that accompanies the treatment of dyspareunia since women receiving placebo treatment in a trial by Everett et al (1992) improved.

Fatigue

All new mothers will suffer some fatigue postpartum, especially in the early days. Lack of sleep and the responsibilities of a new baby, especially if it is the first, all contribute to fatigue. Adequate help and encouraging rest whenever possible should improve matters. However Thompson et al (2002) found that 47% of women they studied reported fatigue six weeks after childbirth, whilst 69% complained of tiredness after six months in a survey by Brown & Lumley (1998).

REFERENCES

Allen R E, Hosker G L, Smith A R B et al 1990 Pelvic floor damage and childbirth: a neurophysiological study. British Journal of Obstetrics and Gynaecology 97:770–779
Boissonnault J S, Kotarinos R K 1988 In: Wilder E (ed) Obstetric and Gynaecologic Physical Therapy. Churchill Livingstone, Edinburgh
Brown S, Lumley J 1998 Maternal health after childbirth: results of an Australian population based survey. British Journal of Obstetrics and Gynaecology 105:156–161
Brunskill P J, Swain J W 1987 Spontaneous fracture of the coccygeal body during the second stage of labour. Journal of Obstetrics and Gynaecology 270–271
Bump R C, Hurt W G, Fantle A et al 1991 Assessment of Kegel pelvic floor muscle exercises performance after brief verbal instruction. American Journal of Obstetrics and Gynecology 165:322–329
Calguneri M, Bird H A, Wright V 1982 Changes in joint laxity occurring during pregnancy. Annals of Rheumatic Disease 41:126–128
Driessen F 1987 Postpartum pelvic arthropathy with unusual features. British Journal of Obstetrics and Gynaecology 94:870–872
Everett T, McIntosh J, Grant A 1992 Ultrasound therapy for persistent postnatal perineal pain and dyspareunia – A randomised placebo-controlled trial. Physiotherapy. 78:263–267
Fry D 1999 Diastasis symphysis pubis. Journal of the Association of Chartered Physiotherapists in Obstetrics and Gynaecology 85:11–18
Gilleard W L, Brown J M M 1996 Structure and function of the abdominal muscles in primigravid subjects during pregnancy and the immediate postbirth period. Physical Therapy 76:750–762
Glazener C, Abdalla M, Stroud P et al 1997 Postnatal morbidity: extent, causes, prevention and treatment. British Journal of Obstetrics and Gynaecology 102:282–287
Grant A, Sleep J, McIntosh J et al 1989 Ultrasound and pulsed electromagnetic energy treatment for perineal trauma. A randomised placebo-controlled trial. British Journal of Obstetrics and Gynaecology 6:434–439
Hay-Smith E J C 2002 Therapeutic ultrasound for postpartum perineal pain and dyspareunia. The Cochrane Library (Issue 1) 2002
Horsley K 1998 Fitness in the childbearing year. In: Sapsford R, Bullock-Saxton J, Markwell S (eds) Women's Health. WB Saunders, London
Kitzinger S, Walters R 1981 Some Women's Experience of Episiotomy. National Childbirth Trust, London
Low J, Reed A 2000 Electrotherapy Explained. Principles and Practice 3rd edn. Butterworth Heinemann, Oxford
MacArthur C, Glazener C M A, Wilson P D et al 2001 Obstetric practice and faecal incontinence three months after delivery. British Journal of Obstetrics and Gynaecology 108:678–683
McIntosh J 1988 Research in reading into treatment of perineal trauma and late dyspareunia. Journal of the Association of Chartered Physiotherapists in Obstetrics and Gynaecology 62:17
McIntosh J M 1993 Incidence of separated symphysis pubis. Midwives Chronicle and Nursing Notes Jan: 23–24
MacLennan A H, Taylor A W, Wilson D H et al 2000 The prevalence of pelvic floor disorders and their relationship to gender, age, parity and mode of delivery. British Journal of Obstetrics and Gynaecology 107:1460–1470

Marshall K, Totterdale D, McConnell D et al 1996 Urinary incontinence and constipation during pregnancy and after childbirth. Physiotherapy 82(2): 98–103

Moore W, James D K 1989 A random trial of three topical analgesic agents in the treatment of episiotomy pain following instrumental vaginal delivery. Journal of Obstetrics and Gynaecology 10:35–39

Mørkved S, Bø K 1999 Prevalence of urinary incontinence during pregnancy and postpartum. International Urogynecology Journal 10:394–398

Noble E 1995 Essential Exercises for the Childbearing Year, 4th edn. New Life Images, Harwich USA

Palastanga N P 1994 Heat and Cold. In: Wells P E, Frampton V, Bowsher D (eds) Pain Management by Physiotherapy 2nd edn. Butterworth Heinemann, Oxford

Polden M, Mantle J 1990 Physiotherapy in Obstetrics and Gynaecology. Butterworth-Heinemann, London

Scriven M W, Jones D A, McKnight L 1995 The importance of pubic pain following childbirth: a clinical and ultrasonographic study of diastasis of the pubic symphysis. Journal of the Royal Society of Medicine 88:28–30

Shepherd A 1980 Re-education of the muscles of the pelvic floor. In: Mandelstam D (ed) Incontinence and its Management. Croom Helm, London

Sleep J M, Grant A, Garcia J et al 1984 West Berkshire perineal management trial. British Medical Journal 289:587–590

Snooks S J, Henry M M, Swash M 1985 Faecal incontinence due to external sphincter division in childbirth is associated with damage to the innervation of the pelvic floor musculature. A double pathology. British Journal of Obstetrics and Gynaecology 92:824–828

Steen M, Cooper K 1998 Cold therapy and perineal wounds: too cool or not too cool? British Journal of Midwifery 6(9):572–579

Steen M, Cooper K, Marchant P et al 2000 A randomized control trial to compare the effectiveness of icepacks and Epifoam with cooling maternity gel packs at alleviating postnatal perineal trauma. Midwifery 16(1):48–55

Sultan A H, Kamm M A, Hudson C H et al 1993 Anal sphincter disruption during vaginal delivery. New England Journal of Medicine 329(26):1905–1911

Swash M 1993 Faecal incontinence, childbirth is responsible for most cases. British Medical Journal 307:636–637

Thompson J F, Roberts C L, Currie M et al 2002 Prevalence and persistence of health problems after childbirth: association with parity and method of birth. Birth 29(2):83–94

Wilson P D, Herbison R M, Herbison G P 1996 Obstetric practice and the prevalence of urinary incontinence three months after delivery. British Journal of Obstetrics and Gynaecology 103:154–161

9

Postnatal exercises and advice

Postnatal exercises following normal
delivery   101
  Circulatory exercises   101
  The pelvic floor   102
  Abdominal exercises   104
  Core trunk stability
    exercises   106
Postnatal exercises following assisted
delivery   109
Postnatal exercises and advice
following caesarean delivery   109

Circulatory exercises   110
Abdominal exercises   111
Pelvic floor exercise   111
Postnatal exercises following
stillbirth or neonatal
death   112
Postnatal care of the back   112
  Daily activities   114
Exercises to avoid   115
Postnatal classes   115
References   116

This chapter includes early exercises and advice following normal, assisted and caesarean delivery.

Following delivery, the new mother's body begins its recovery and gradually returns to the pre-pregnancy state. Some rest and postnatal exercise will help this physiological process to take place smoothly. It is of advantage if the mother has had the opportunity to consider postnatal exercises prior to delivery. Although she may be suffering from fatigue, discomfort and the responsibilities of mothering, the subject should be broached positively and the following simple exercises encouraged.

POSTNATAL EXERCISES FOLLOWING NORMAL DELIVERY

Circulatory exercises

These exercises should be performed as often as possible after delivery. They are intended to maintain and/or improve the mother's circulation in the immediate post-partum period when she could be at risk of deep venous thrombosis or other circulatory complications. The exercises may be done on the bed several times every waking hour and should be continued until the mother is fully mobile and there is no ankle oedema present. They are especially relevant after an epidural anaesthesia when there may be considerable oedema of feet and ankles and the circulation is sluggish. Early ambulation should prevent deep venous thrombosis.

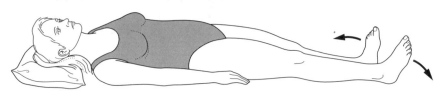

Figure 9.1 Foot exercises.

Foot Exercises (Figure 9.1)

- Sit or lie with the knees straight. Bend and stretch the ankles briskly at least 12 times, emphasising dorsiflexion rather than plantarflexion to avoid cramp. Keeping the knees and hips still, circle both ankles in as big a circle as possible at least 12 times in each direction.

Leg tightening

- Sit or lie with the legs straight. Pull both feet upwards at the ankle and press the back of the knees down onto the bed. Hold this position for a count of 5, breathing normally, then relax. Repeat 10 times.

Deep breathing

Diaphragmatic breathing helps the venous return through the pumping action of the diaphragm on the inferior vena cava and should be repeated several times a day until the mother is fully mobile.

- In any position, take 3 or 4 (no more) deep breaths to encourage full ventilation of the lungs.

Previous advice given antenatally, i.e. to avoid prolonged standing and sitting or lying with legs crossed applies postnatally. Encourage the mother to lie down to rest when possible. Circulatory exercises are helpful at all times but, once the mother is up and about, there are more important exercises to practise if her time is limited.

The pelvic floor

Pelvic-floor exercises will strengthen the pelvic-floor muscles postnatally with the aim of regaining their full function as soon as possible and helping to prevent any long-term urinary problems or prolapse. However, contraction and relaxation of these muscles will also assist in relieving any discomfort in the perineum, which may be present as a result of delivery, and aid healing by promoting local circulation and reducing oedema. Pelvic floor exercises should be started as soon as possible following delivery to prevent loss of cortical control over the muscles due to perineal pain and apprehension about damaging stitches (Shepherd, 1980). The mother who has had an episiotomy following epidural anaesthesia may feel a sudden intense perineal pain after a painless labour. She may need pain relief to prevent inhibition of the pelvic-floor contraction (see Ch. 7); all mothers must be encouraged to contract their pelvic floor muscles little and often, slowly and quickly, in the early postpartum period. Postnatally the woman may find the pelvic-floor exercise more difficult because of stretching at delivery and possible discomfort from a bruised or sutured perineum. Plenty of reassurance will be needed as she will probably find she cannot reach the number of contractions she achieved antenatally.

Pelvic floor exercise

- Close the back passage as though preventing a bowel action, squeeze the middle and front passages too as though preventing the flow of urine, then lift up all three passages inside. Hold strongly for as long as possible up to 10 seconds, breathing normally throughout. Relax and rest for three seconds. Repeat the above slowly as many times as possible up to a maximum of 10.

Repeat the exercise lifting and letting go more quickly up to 10 times without holding the contraction. The number of repetitions will build up gradually as women will only manage a few initially but must be reassured that this is normal.

By exercising these muscles slowly and quickly, both the slow-twitch type I and the fast-twitch type II muscle fibres will be strengthened (Gilpin et al 1989). The performance of the pelvic-floor exercise can be memory-linked to activities associated with the baby, for example, feeding, bathing, washing. It can be practised whilst sitting on the lavatory after each bladder-emptying. This is a relaxed position in which to contract these muscles. A notice can be placed behind the hospital toilet doors as a further reminder. If a painful perineum makes the exercise difficult when sitting, it could be practised in prone-lying, or side-lying with a pillow between the legs, or standing with legs slightly apart.

Advice should be given to brace the pelvic floor when coughing, laughing, lifting or squatting down. Mothers should be warned that it could take up to three months to regain full pelvic-floor function. However, all women should be encouraged to continue with regular pelvic-floor exercises for the rest of their lives to help prevent future urinary problems (see Ch. 3). They can test the functional strength of their pelvic-floor muscles 8–12 weeks post delivery by jumping up and down with a full bladder and coughing deeply two or three times while doing so. There should not be any leakage of urine if the muscles have regained their former strength and function. If leakage does occur on testing, the pelvic-floor muscles need further intensive exercising and retesting four weeks later. If there is still leakage, the mother should be referred to a women's health physiotherapist for specialist treatment. In some areas women may self-refer within 12 weeks of delivery, otherwise they will need a doctor's referral for specialist physiotherapy. Subsequent pregnancies will only subject the pelvic floor to further strain and should not be undertaken before rehabilitation of the pelvic floor is complete.

Abdominal exercises

During pregnancy the abdominal corset has stretched until at term it is approximately twice its original length. All the abdominal muscles will need exercising to regain their former length and strength but the most important muscle because of its role in pelvic stability is transversus. Working the rectus muscle strongly by performing straight or oblique curl-ups is inadvisable until transversus abdominis is working efficiently to stabilize the pelvis. The transversus exercise may be started whenever the woman feels able and should be encouraged frequently whilst she is doing activities with the baby.

Transversus exercise (Figure 9.2)

- Lie on the back with the knees bent and the feet flat on the bed. Place hands over the lower abdomen in front of the hips. Breathe in and at the end of the outward breath pull in the lower part of the abdomen below the umbilicus and hold for a count of up to 10, continuing to breathe normally. Repeat up to 10 times.

This should be a gentle contraction only to encourage the type I slow twitch fibres which assist in the stability of the pelvis. It is easy to do in conjunction with other activities and can be performed frequently in many positions, for example, side-lying, sitting or standing. The pregnancy starting position of prone kneeling should not be used whilst there is any

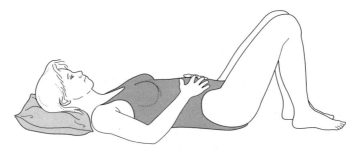

Figure 9.2 Transversus exercise.

ıere is a remote possibility of an air embolus entering the raw
(Horsley 1998). Because of this, it is advisable to avoid this
ɔur to six weeks postpartum.

ɪnancy, the transversus and pelvic floor muscles will work
and this should be encouraged to improve pelvic stability.

us and pelvic floor exercise

ɪɪɪc acuɔɪɪs of both the transversus and the pelvic floor muscles will be
enhanced by combining the two exercises (Sapsford et al 2001). This
co-activation will be particularly beneficial postnatally especially if a
pelvic floor muscle contraction is difficult to initiate. The woman can try to
work transversus then bring in a pelvic floor contraction or vice versa. It is
important to use this combined contraction functionally during activities
to protect the spine and pelvic joints. A new mother has many tasks to perform which involve lifting, for example, changing baby's nappy, putting
baby into the cot, feeding. She should be reminded to use transversus and
the pelvic floor muscles before starting to do any of these tasks.

Pelvic tilting (Figure 9.3)

The pelvic tilting exercise can be performed early in the postpartum
period and is particularly useful if the mother has any postural backache.

- Lie on the back with the knees bent and the feet flat on the surface. Pull
  in the abdominal muscles, tighten the muscles of the buttocks and press
  the small of the back down onto the surface. Hold the position for a
  count of 5, breathing normally, then relax. Repeat five times, building
  up to 10 or more repetitions over the following weeks. Repeat the
  exercise more rhythmically (pelvic rocking) to help to relieve any
  postural stiffness or backache that may be present following delivery.

It can be done in several positions, for instance, sitting and standing may be more convenient than lying when the mother is at home
and busy.

Rectus check

About the third day the rectus muscles should be checked to exclude any
excessive diastasis (see Ch. 3). The oblique muscles are inserted diagonally
into the linea alba and rectus sheath (see Ch. 1) and any gap between the
rectus bellies could increase when the obliques are contracted (Noble
1995). Up to 2.5 cm (2 fingers) width between the rectus muscles is considered acceptable at this stage. If the gap is greater than this, stronger

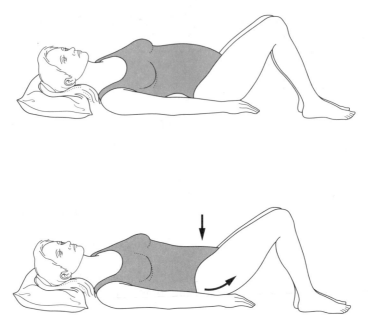

Figure 9.3 Pelvic tilting exercise.

abdominal exercises or rotation should not be performed as the stress on the linea alba may increase the separation.

The midwife is the ideal person to check for diastasis when she is palpating the fundus. The mother should lie on her back with one pillow under her head, knees bent up and feet flat on the bed. With the midwife's fingers pressed into the abdomen either just above or below the umbilicus, the mother is asked to lift her head and shoulders off the pillow towards her knees. The rectus muscles will be felt taut either side of the fingers if there is no diastasis. If the rectus muscles cannot be felt until two or more fingers are inserted and peaking of the recti is apparent, only transversus and pelvic tilting exercises should be commenced and practised several times a day (see Ch. 3). After a few days the rectus check can be repeated. If the gap is significant and is not reducing, the woman should be referred to a woman's health physiotherapist (see Ch. 3).

Core trunk stability exercises

To encourage transversus to stabilize the pelvis while movements of the lower limb are performed, the following exercises may be introduced about 5–10 days after a normal delivery if there are no musculoskeletal pelvic problems.

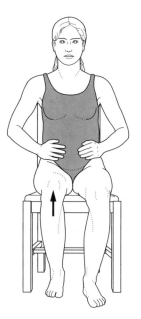

Figure 9.4 Core stability exercise.

- In sitting with feet flat on the floor and hands over the lower abdominal muscles, draw in the transversus and pelvic floor muscles and raise one knee so the foot is a couple of inches off the floor. Hold for up to five seconds making sure the pelvis and spine remain level. Repeat five times with each leg (Figure 9.4). Gradually increase the hold to 10 seconds and repeat 10 times.

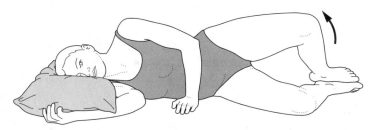

Figure 9.5 Core stability exercise – knee raising.

- In side lying with both knees bent up in front, draw in transversus and the pelvic floor and lift the top knee by turning the hip outwards whilst keeping the heels together. Hold for up to five seconds making sure the pelvis or spine do not rotate. Repeat five times with each leg (Figure 9.5). Gradually increase the hold to 10 seconds and repeat 10 times.

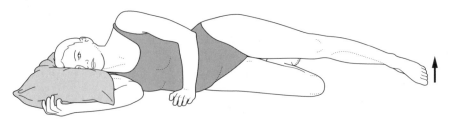

Figure 9.6 Hip abduction in side-lying.

- In side-lying with the underneath knee bent backwards, draw in the lower abdomen and raise the top leg up towards the ceiling keeping it in line with the body. Hold for up to five seconds making sure the back and pelvis do not rotate. Repeat five times with each leg (Figure 9.6). Gradually increase the hold to 10 seconds and repeat 10 times. Over the next few weeks progress to controlling the pelvis and spine whilst lifting the leg towards the ceiling with the hip rotated outwards.

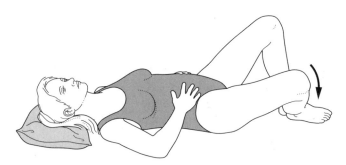

Figure 9.7 Allowing knee to roll outwards whilst keeping pelvis still.

- In back-lying with knees bent up and feet flat on the floor. Place hands over the front of the hips, pull in the lower abdomen and let the right knee lower outwards slightly controlling it to make sure that the pelvis stay level and the back stays flat. Slowly return the knee to the upright position. Repeat five times with alternate knees (Figure 9.7). Gradually increase repetitions up to 10. Over the next few weeks, progress to controlling the pelvis as the knee is lowered further.

- In back-lying with knees bent up and feet flat on the floor. Place hands in front of the hips, pull in the lower abdomen and gently slide the heel of one leg downwards keeping the back flat and the pelvis level. Stop if the pelvis starts to move. Slowly return the knee to the bent position. Repeat five times with alternate legs (Figure 9.8). Gradually increase

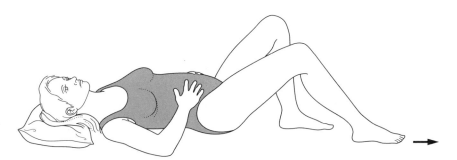

Figure 9.8 Straightening one leg whilst keeping the pelvis and back still.

repetitions up to 10. Over the next few weeks, progress to controlling the pelvis whilst straightening the leg further.

All the exercises will be more effective if performed slowly and the number of repetitions increased gradually according to individual capabilities. It is always better to exercise little and often rather than just once a day. However if the mother is feeling tired or unwell, she should be guided by her body and defer the exercises until she feels better. Other exercises should be left until pelvic stability has been re-established.

POSTNATAL EXERCISES FOLLOWING ASSISTED DELIVERY

Mothers who have undergone a forceps delivery or ventouse extraction will have sutures and may have bruising and oedema. These mothers may be reluctant to exercise, but should be encouraged to perform the circulatory exercises (especially if they have had epidural anaesthesia) and gentle pelvic floor exercises which will aid healing of the perineum. The transversus exercise should be introduced whenever the mother feels up to it.

Comfortable resting positions are side-lying with a pillow between the legs (see Figure 9.9) and prone-lying (many mothers forget they can now lie on their front) with one pillow under the hips and another under the head and shoulders (Figure 9.10). Breastfeeding may be more comfortable in a side-lying rather than a sitting position.

POSTNATAL EXERCISES AND ADVICE FOLLOWING CAESAREAN DELIVERY

The mother should be taught how to move up and down the bed by bending her knees, pulling in her abdominal muscles and curling forwards whilst pushing on her hands and feet. She will be able to move her body in a forwards or backwards direction. She should not attempt to sit up

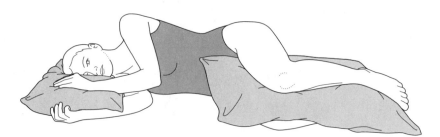

Figure 9.9 Comfortable position in side-lying.

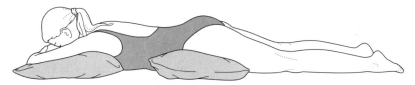

Figure 9.10 Prone-lying with pillow under hips.

forwards from a lying position, but instead continue to roll over onto her side as described in Chapter 3. This is also the easiest way of getting out of bed – tightening transversus and pushing up into a sitting position over the edge of the bed.

Flatulence is often the cause of great discomfort post-delivery, and may be relieved by gently rolling the knees a few inches to each side (in a tic-toc action). **NB.** The knees should not be taken far to the sides in case any diastasis of recti is present.

Deep breathing followed by huffing (short forced expirations) will help to loosen any secretions in the lungs that may be present after a general anaesthetic. If the mother needs to cough, she should bend her knees and support her wound with her hands or a pillow, whilst leaning forwards or sitting over the edge of the bed (see Figure 9.11). This will prevent undue strain on the sutures, increase her confidence and reduce pain.

Circulatory exercises

Vigorous foot and leg exercises for the circulation are extremely important following caesarean delivery especially if this has been performed under epidural anaesthesia. She will have been given extra fluids and her legs will feel heavy so she must be encouraged to do these exercises very regularly during the first couple of days. Three or four deep breaths after the foot and leg exercises will also help the circulation whilst the mother is relatively immobile.

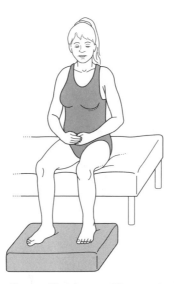

Figure 9.11 Supporting position for coughing, post-caesarean delivery.

Abdominal exercises

Transversus should be exercised as soon as the mother feels up to it. She should be encouraged to tighten her transversus before doing any activities with the baby and if she needs to cough. If the mother has any postural backache resulting from the tilted position on the operating table and the epidural numbness (see Ch. 3), she may find it soothing to perform the pelvic tilting exercises rhythmically as a rocking action to ease the discomfort.

A check for diastasis of the recti can be done when the mother feels comfortable probably after seven days or so. Progression of the core stability exercises described following a normal delivery should be slower than that following a normal delivery and prone-lying will not be a comfortable position for some time.

Pelvic floor exercise

Pelvic floor exercises are still important following a caesarean delivery, though if a catheter is in situ, only an occasional contraction should be tried before its removal. It has been demonstrated that it is the pregnancy rather than the delivery that causes the greatest strain on the pelvic floor muscles (Francis 1960) and that caesarean delivery is not associated with a significant reduction in long-term pelvic floor morbidity compared with vaginal delivery (MacLennan et al 2000). The author has treated several women suffering from urinary problems who have undergone caesarean births only.

POSTNATAL EXERCISES FOLLOWING STILLBIRTH OR NEONATAL DEATH

Women who have had the sad experience of a stillbirth or neonatal death, or who have a very ill baby may be cared for in a single room and tend to miss out on postnatal exercises. Special effort needs to be made to offer these women exercises and advice about normal daily activities. They usually prefer to be given this on a one to one basis. A sensitive leaflet should be available which does not refer to the baby, for example, feeding, nappy changing. These women may be going back to work earlier than they had previously planned and need advice on re-educating their abdominal and pelvic floor muscles, especially when performing functional activities. They may appreciate a follow-up appointment with a physiotherapist after a few weeks as it is obviously inappropriate for them to attend a postnatal reunion class.

POSTNATAL CARE OF THE BACK

During the early postnatal period the mother's joints are still unstable because of the hormonal influence on the ligaments and can remain so for up to six months (Polden & Mantle 1990). The abdominal muscles, which help to support the spine and control the pelvic tilt, are stretched and weak. So the new mother is at her most vulnerable just when she is faced with so many new activities for the baby that involve bending, stooping or lifting. She is looking forward to being able to resume normal activities and rarely considers possible long-term problems. It is extremely important that the midwife explains the underlying anatomy and physiology to the mother and teaches and/or reinforces awareness of good back care both in hospital and more especially at home. The midwife has the opportunity, when with the mother, to discuss positions for changing and bathing baby that avoid stooping and carrying heavy baths of water. Both standing at a surface that is at waist height, or kneeling at a surface which is coffee-table height obviate the need for stooping whilst carrying out tasks for the baby. The midwife can suggest comfortable and supported positions in which to feed baby so the mother is not bending forward (see Figure 9.12).

Correct posture in all positions will not only alleviate backache, but should also give the mother a sense of good body-image. At first, it will be a matter of re-educating her postural sense in front of a full-length mirror as the brain has got used to the pregnant stance. If she stands sideways to the mirror she will soon see whether her outline is still a semi-pregnant one! However, if the mother checks her posture and braces transversus whenever she stands up, it will soon become a good habit.

Lifting must be kept to an absolute minimum for the first few weeks if this is at all possible. This is the advice that would be given to a patient

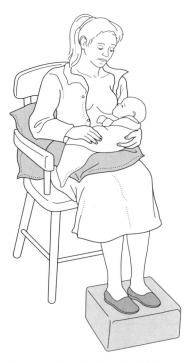

Figure 9.12 Positions for feeding.

with back problems, but it is also relevant in order to prevent problems in someone with stretched ligaments and muscles. However a mother may have to lift if there is no one else to do it for her. In this case she should be encouraged to make the object handled as light as possible and hold it close to the body. With a little planning, some lifting may be delegated to others. If the mother has no help, the correct lifting procedures as described in Chapter 4 must be followed to avoid back strain at this very vulnerable time. Toddlers should be encouraged to climb onto a chair instead of being lifted, or onto the second or third stair for dressing to avoid the mother stooping (see Figure 9.13).

Relatives may need reminding that the newly-delivered mother needs adequate rest and relaxation periods at home as well as time to do her postnatal exercises. More mothers are having their babies by caesarean delivery and many relatives do not appreciate the fact that these mothers have undergone major surgery and will require even more rest and support at home. The midwife will probably find herself answering many questions about when the mother can resume normal activities after caesarean delivery. Driving is a popular topic and the mother should be advised to check with her insurance company that she is fully covered.

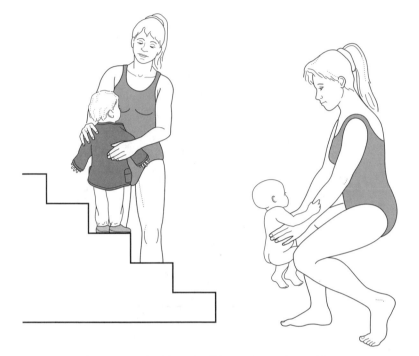

Figure 9.13 Positions for lifting and dressing toddler.

When to start also depends on her rate of recovery as she must be able to concentrate fully, be able to twist round comfortably and be able to perform an emergency stop.

Daily activities

Heavy housework, for example, vacuuming, moving furniture, cleaning windows should be avoided for several weeks after delivery to prevent back strain. Walking, cycling and swimming are good ways of supplementing the above postnatal exercises, but more strenuous keep-fit classes, aerobics or competitive sports should be left for at least ten to twelve weeks. Prior to this, mothers may join especially designed exercise-to-music or aquanatal classes from six to eight weeks (see Ch. 12), if they are run by qualified personnel. If any joints are still affected by the hormonal influence on the ligaments or if there are any urinary problems, more strenuous exercise should be avoided until these are completely resolved. New activities need to be started gently and built up gradually.

EXERCISES TO AVOID

Two commonly practised 'abdominal exercises' are double-leg raising and sit-ups with straight legs. These are high-risk exercises for anyone to perform and may result in compression injury to vertebral discs or muscle and ligament damage (Donovan et al 1988). There are added risks to the postnatal woman because of stretched muscles and lax ligaments (see Ch. 7).

NB. These two exercises should never be performed (see Figure 9.14).

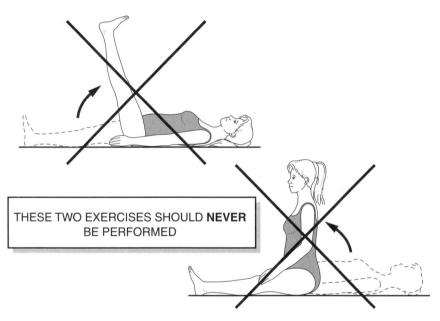

THESE TWO EXERCISES SHOULD **NEVER** BE PERFORMED

Figure 9.14   These two exercises should *never* be performed.

POSTNATAL CLASSES

Ideally, mothers should be taught the postnatal exercises in the antenatal period and encouraged to start them as soon as possible in the postnatal period. Unfortunately, many mothers do not attend antenatal classes and will need individually-supervised tuition postnatally. It is very beneficial if group exercises are performed on the postnatal wards, but with early discharges this is practically impossible to arrange. Most midwives will find they are teaching postnatal exercises on a one-to-one basis especially in the home. However, a compromise might be for a postnatal exercise class to be held in the community, which mothers could attend when they wished (see Ch. 11). Exercises at these classes could be progressed to include more work for the stabilizing muscles of the pelvis in preparation for rejoining aerobic classes and more strenuous sporting activities. The sessions would provide a support network for new mothers and an opportunity for professionals to pick up problems.

REFERENCES

Donovan G, McNamara J, Gianoli P 1988 Exercise Danger. Wellness Australia Pty Ltd, Western Australia
Francis W 1960 The onset of stress incontinence. Journal of Obstetrics and Gynaecology of the British Empire 67:899–903
Gilpin S A, Gosling A, Smith A R B, Warrell D W 1989 The pathogenesis of genitourinary prolapse and stress incontinence of urine. A histological and histochemical study. British Journal of Obstetrics and Gynaecology 96:15–23
Horsley K 1998 Fitness in the childbearing years In: Sapsford R, Bullock-Saxton J, Markwell, S (eds) Women's Health. WB Saunders, London
MacLennan A H, Taylor A W, Wilson D H et al 2000 The prevalence of pelvic floor disorders and their relevance to gender, age, parity and mode of delivery. British Journal of Obstetrics and Gynaecology 107(12):1460–1470
Noble B 1995 Essential Exercises for the Childbearing Year 3rd edn. Houghton Mifflin, Boston
Polden M, Mantle J 1990 Physiotherapy in Obstetrics and Gynaecology. Butterworth-Heinemann, Oxford
Sapsford R R, Hodges P W, Richardson C A et al 2001 Co-activation of the abdominal and pelvic floor muscles during voluntary exercises. Neurology and Urodynamics 20:31–42
Shepherd A 1980 Re-education of the muscles of the pelvic floor. In: Mandelstam D (ed) Incontinence and its Management. Croom Helm, London

10

Teaching exercises

Facilities and equipment   118
Arranging the group   118
Teaching exercises to others   120
Antenatal exercise instructions and
   information   120
   Foot and leg exercises   120
   Pelvic floor exercise   121
   Abdominal exercises   122
   Transversus   122
   Pelvic tilting   124
Postnatal exercise instructions and
   information   127
   Foot and leg exercises   127

Pelvic-floor exercise   128
Abdominal exercises   129
Transversus   130
Pelvic tilting   131
Core trunk stability
   exercises   134
Evaluation of teaching   137
Additional antenatal exercises   137
   Shoulder, arm and chest
      exercises   137
   Stretching exercises   138
Warning   141
Further advice   142

This chapter addresses the important facts to consider when teaching exercises. It includes the instructions for antenatal and postnatal exercises in different starting positions together with the necessary teaching points.

Physiotherapists specialise in teaching physical skills. It is therefore more difficult for other professionals who are not specifically trained in this field to teach exercises. It is essential that before embarking on this undertaking, the prospective teacher should follow simple guidelines.

She should:

- be proficient at performing the exercises or skills herself
- be completely familiar with the terminology of each exercise or skill
- be able to recognize signs of muscle fatigue
- practise teaching one or two willing colleagues or family members unfamiliar with the skills
- ask for feedback before attempting to teach a larger group of women/partners.

Several points should be observed when teaching physical skills. The group participants need to know:

- why they are learning the particular exercise and what the benefits are
- how to perform the exercise correctly
- why it is necessary to stop if not performing the exercise correctly
- when, where, how often and how many times to practise the exercise
- any additional relevant information and advice.

The teacher must be aware of recognizing signs of muscle fatigue, i.e. any aching in the muscles, inappropriate recruitment of other muscle groups ('cheating'), shaking muscles or straining during the exercise. Exercises should be progressed very gently at each individual's rate.

It must be remembered that in any group one or two members may have physical problems, for example, lumbar disc lesion, asthma, congenital abnormalities, which could be exacerbated by some exercises or postures. No discomfort should be experienced whilst performing any exercise and the group should be reassured that it is quite permissible to omit a particular exercise or adopt an alternative position if uncomfortable.

FACILITIES AND EQUIPMENT

Many teachers will find themselves with less than perfect facilities in crowded community clinics. Ideally, the room selected for exercise classes should be private, well ventilated, have plenty of floor and wall space, lighting which can be dimmed, and be close to toilets and refreshment facilities. Chairs of different heights and types would allow posture to be demonstrated in several positions and provide an alternative for the woman who is not comfortable on the floor. A full-length mirror is important to check correct posture in standing. Mats are desirable but not essential if the room is carpeted. For the exercise and relaxation sessions, each woman should have a right-angled wedge which can be either upright against the wall as a backrest for exercises in sitting, or on the floor to allow the woman to be at an angle of 45 degrees when half-lying. In addition three pillows would permit her to practise relaxation in different positions. However, pillows can be doubled over, upturned chairs can be used as backrests and women with their own transport are usually willing to bring pillows from home. Failing all of the above suggestions, it may only be possible to demonstrate alternative positions for some activities.

ARRANGING THE GROUP

Ideally, the group should be arranged in a semi-circle or horseshoe so all members can see each other and the educator. Each woman will then feel part of the group and exercises can be checked easily. The teacher should have eye contact with each member of the group whenever possible. The women will feel less threatened if the teacher is at the same level as themselves, i.e. on the floor or on a beanbag rather than standing, though it may be necessary and desirable to move around from time to time. The group should also be encouraged to change position frequently. The following points will be useful to consider when teaching exercises to a group (see Box 10.1).

Box 10.1 Teaching exercises

- select appropriate starting position
- clearly describe and/or demonstrate each exercise
- state number of repetitions
- state how often to practise
- advise how to progress each exercise
- check each individual is performing correctly
- check for signs of muscle fatigue
- encourage practice at home
- add relevant information and advice.

The most appropriate starting position for each exercise should be selected and the reasons explained to the group. Many exercises can be executed in alternative positions to suit individual needs or to progress the exercise. The exercises should be introduced one at a time and described very clearly using phraseology suitable to the group and/or demonstrated before the participants are asked to adopt the starting position. It is not easy to see or hear the instructions when lying down.

Individuals should be aware of the optimum number of repetitions, how frequently to repeat and how to progress each exercise. The group should be encouraged to practise regularly at home. Memory-links to suit individuals could be suggested in discussion. The members of the group should be individually checked to ensure the exercise is being performed correctly and that there are no signs of muscle fatigue. If the performance is incorrect and allowed to pass unchecked, the woman could cause problems for herself if she continued to practise. Sensitivity must be used to avoid embarrassment to any individual, so a general comment is preferable, though personal correction may still be required.

For easy reference, all the exercises described in the antenatal sections are repeated in the postnatal section with the relevant information that should be given to the learner. The number of repetitions is only approximate for the group as a whole. At all times women should be encouraged to listen to their own bodies and alter the repetitions accordingly to avoid muscle fatigue.

Sometimes the exercises will be taught just to one woman on her own. Although there will not be the added enjoyment of a group situation, some women prefer this; the explanation being tailored to the woman's individual needs. There will also be women with special needs where exercises may have to be adapted. It may be that all exercise has to be performed in a chair rather than using a mat, or that only part of the routine can be utilised. Often the woman (and partner) will need individual sessions to reinforce the teaching of the exercises but could attend the group as well for support.

The use of music can help to motivate and increase enjoyment and interest in exercise sessions. It can be used with the basic exercises taught both antenatally in preparation for parenthood classes (Ch. 4), and postnatally (Ch. 9). Music with or without beats can be used and classical music is often appropriate. Music should not control and dominate the exercises and it is acceptable to allow pauses during performance when teaching points, instructions and information are given. The teacher will need to emphasise correct execution as the women may be listening to the music and not concentrating on the exercise. During the relaxation period, well-chosen music will help to create a peaceful atmosphere. Music must always be used with care so that a high standard of exercise performance is maintained.

TEACHING EXERCISES TO OTHERS

The reader must check that she is fully cognisant of the contents of Chapters 4 and 9 and have confidence in her own performance of each physical skill. She should now be ready to try out the following exercises on three or four willing colleagues or friends, using the information and instructions on the following pages.

ANTENATAL EXERCISE INSTRUCTIONS AND INFORMATION

Foot and leg exercises

Aim of exercises:

To improve the circulation, particularly the venous return.

Why necessary:

Circulation is slowed because of the hormonal influence on vein walls, increased blood volume, and pressure from the enlarged uterus. Sluggish circulation could lead to cramp, swollen ankles and varicose veins.

Starting position:

Sitting on the bed, floor or on a chair with the legs stretched out in front and supported.

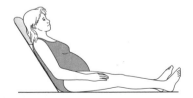

Figure 10.1   Starting position: sitting.

Foot Exercises

- Bend and stretch the ankles briskly. Repeat at least 12 times.
- Circle both feet in as large a circle as possible, keeping the knees still. Repeat at least 12 times in each direction.

Leg tightening

- Pull both feet upwards at the ankle and press the back of the knees down onto the surface. Hold for a count of 5, breathing normally, then relax. Repeat 10 times.

Frequency:

Whenever possible, particularly early morning, late evening, and when sitting with legs elevated.

Advice:

- sit with legs elevated and supported
- sit instead of standing when possible
- wriggle toes when standing
- do not sit or lie with legs crossed
- wear support tights if necessary
- wear appropriate footwear (see Ch. 4)
- change position frequently
- walking aids circulation.

Pelvic floor exercise

Aim of exercise:

To promote awareness and tone the muscles for pregnancy, labour and the puerperium.

Why necessary:

There is strain on the pelvic floor because of the hormonal influence on fascia and muscle, the extra weight of the pregnancy and the delivery. Weak muscles could lead to urinary problems, prolapse and sexual problems.

Starting position:

Any comfortable position with the legs slightly apart.

The exercise

- Squeeze the back passage as though preventing a bowel action, squeeze the middle and front passages too as though preventing the flow of urine, then lift up all three passages inside. Hold strongly for as long as possible up to 10 seconds, breathing normally throughout. Relax and rest for three seconds. Repeat the above slowly as many times as possible up to a maximum of 10 times. Repeat the exercise, lifting up and letting go more quickly up to 10 times without holding the contraction.

NB. Make sure you do not tighten the thigh or buttock muscles.

Frequency:

As many occasions as possible so it becomes a habit. Use a memory-link, for example, after each bladder emptying. Very occasionally test by a midstream stop.

Advice:

- get into the habit of doing the exercise anywhere, any time
- stop midstream only occasionally
- do not hold breath
- do not tighten thighs or buttocks
- contract slowly first, then quickly
- refer for professional advice if necessary.

Abdominal exercises:

Aim of exercises:

To tone the natural abdominal corset, maintain pelvic stability and prevent and relieve backache.

Why necessary:

The abdominal muscles are weakened by the hormonal effect on muscle and fascia and the stretching during pregnancy. Altered posture and pelvic instability may lead to back pain during pregnancy and after. Transversus is the core stability muscle and is vital to regaining core trunk stability.

Transversus

Starting position – prone kneeling:

Kneeling on all fours with the arms and thighs vertical, hands directly under shoulders and knees directly under hips.

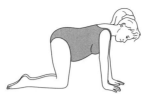

Figure 10.2 Starting position: prone-kneeling.

The exercise

- Keeping the spine in the mid position, breathe in and whilst breathing out gently draw up the lower abdominal muscles towards the spine. Hold this position for up to 10 seconds, continuing to breathe normally, then relax slowly. Repeat up to 10 times.

Starting position – side-lying:

Lying on one side with both knees bent up and a pillow between the legs.

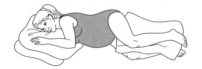

Figure 10.3 Starting position: side-lying.

The exercise

- Keeping the spine in the mid position, breathe in and whilst breathing out, gently draw in the lower abdominal muscles towards the spine. Hold this position for up to 10 seconds, continuing to breathe normally, then relax slowly. Repeat up to 10 times.

Starting position – sitting:

Sitting well back on a dining-type chair with the feet on the floor. Place hands on the abdomen below the umbilicus with the fingers towards midline.

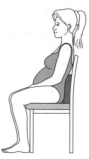

Figure 10.4 Starting position: sitting.

The exercise

• Keeping the spine in the mid position, breathe in and whilst breathing out gently draw in the lower abdominal muscles away from the fingers towards the spine. Hold this position for up to 10 seconds, continuing to breathe normally, then relax slowly. Repeat up to 10 times.

Starting position – standing:

Standing with the weight evenly on both feet.

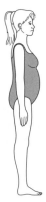

Figure 10.5   Starting position: standing.

The exercise

• Keeping the spine in the mid position, breathe in and whilst breathing out gently draw in the lower abdominal muscles towards the spine. Hold this position for up to 10 seconds, continuing to breathe normally, then relax slowly. Repeat up to 10 times.

Frequency:

Several times a day in any of the different positions. Transversus and the pelvic floor should be co-activated before performing activities such as changing positions, climbing stairs, moving and handling objects and whenever standing for any length of time.

Pelvic tilting

Starting position – half-lying:

Half-lying at an angle of 45 degrees, supported with a wedge and pillows, with the knees bent up and the feet flat on the surface.

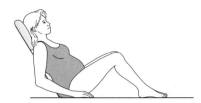

Figure 10.6   Starting position: half-lying.

The exercise

- Pull in the abdominal muscles, tighten the buttock muscles and press the small of the back down onto the support. Hold for a count of 5, breathing normally, then relax. Repeat up to 10 times.

Can also be done more rhythmically without holding the contraction to ease tension in the back whenever necessary.

Starting position – supported sitting:

Sitting well back on a dining-type chair with the hands on the abdomen.

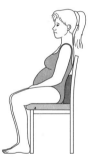

Figure 10.7   Starting position: sitting.

The exercise

- Pull in the abdominals, tighten the buttock muscles and press the small of the back into the back of the chair. Hold for a count of 5, breathing normally, then relax. Repeat up 10 times.

Starting position – reverse sitting:

Sitting the opposite way round on a chair with the arms round the back of the chair.

The exercise

- Pull in the abdominals, tighten the buttock muscles, slightly rounding the lower back, and hold for a count of 5, breathing normally, then relax. Repeat up to 10 times.

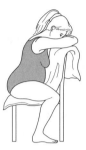

Figure 10.8   Starting position: reverse sitting.

Starting position – standing:

Standing tall with the feet several inches apart and the knees slightly bent.

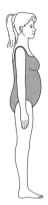

Figure 10.9   Starting position: standing.

The exercise

• Pull in the abdominal muscles, and tuck in the buttocks. Hold for a count of 5, breathing normally, then relax. Repeat up to 10 times.

Starting position – prone kneeling:

Kneeling on all fours with the arms and thighs vertical, hands directly under shoulders and knees directly under hips.

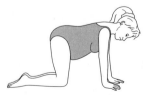

Figure 10.10   Starting position: prone-kneeling.

The exercise

- Pull up the abdominals, tighten the buttock muscles and push the small of the back upwards. Hold for a count of 5, breathing normally, then gently relax the abdominals and allow the spine to flatten – not hollow. Repeat up to 10 times.

Frequency:

Several times a day in the different positions.

Advice:

- when performing any functional activities, for example, changing positions, moving and handling objects, brace both transversus and the pelvic floor to protect the pelvis and spine
- when standing, gently pull in transversus and the pelvic floor muscles
- pelvic tilting exercises can also be performed rhythmically (rocking) to relieve backache
- correct standing posture using mirror
- always distribute weight evenly on both sides of the body when sitting or standing
- refer to a women's health physiotherapist if there are persistent back problems.

POSTNATAL EXERCISE INSTRUCTIONS AND INFORMATION

Foot and leg exercises

Aim of exercises:

To improve the circulation, particularly venous return.

Why necessary:

Circulation is slowed, especially after epidural or general anaesthesia, because of the hormonal influences of pregnancy, loss of fluid at delivery, increased waste products, decreased intra-abdominal pressure and relative immobility. Slowed circulation could lead to deep venous thrombosis, swollen ankles, pulmonary embolus or discomfort in leg.

Starting position:

Lying or sitting on the bed, floor or chair with the legs stretched out in front and supported.

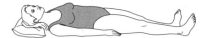

Figure 10.11 Starting position: lying.

Foot Exercises

- Bend and stretch the ankles briskly. Repeat at least 12 times.
- Circle both feet in as large a circle as possible, keeping the knees still. Repeat at least 12 times in each direction.

Leg tightening

- Pull both feet upwards at the ankle and press the back of the knees down onto the surface. Hold for a count of 5, breathing normally, then relax. Repeat 10 times.

Frequency:

Whenever possible, particularly early morning, late evening, and when sitting with the legs elevated.

Advice:

- sit with legs elevated and supported
- sit instead of standing when possible
- wriggle toes when standing
- do not sit or lie with legs crossed
- change position frequently
- walking aids deep venous circulation.

Pelvic-floor exercise

Aim of exercise:

To re-educate and strengthen the muscles and promote healing.

Why necessary:

The weakening of the pelvic floor by the strain of pregnancy or trauma of delivery can lead to urinary and sexual problems and prolapse.

Starting position:

Any comfortable position with legs slightly apart.

The exercise

- Squeeze the back passage as though preventing a bowel action, squeeze the middle and front passages too as though preventing the flow of urine, then lift up all three passages inside. Hold strongly for as long as possible up to a maximum of 10 seconds, breathing normally throughout. Relax and rest for three seconds. Repeat the above slowly as many times as you can up to a maximum of 10. Repeat the exercise, lifting up and letting go more quickly up to 10 times without holding the contraction.

NB. Make sure you do not tighten the thigh or buttock muscles.

Frequency:

As many occasions as possible so it becomes a habit. Use a memory-link, for example, after each bladder emptying. Very occasionally test by a 'midstream stop'. Link the pelvic-floor exercise to activities with the baby.

Advice:

- get into the habit – anywhere, any time
- brace pelvic floor and transversus before performing functional activities
- stop midstream only occasionally
- do not hold breath
- do not tighten thighs or buttocks
- contract slowly first, then quickly
- test strength at 8–12 weeks (see Ch. 9)
- refer to a women's health physiotherapist for advice if necessary.

Abdominal exercises

Aim of exercises:

To strengthen the abdominal muscles and regain full function of the natural muscular corset. Transversus in particular will help to re-establish pelvic stability.

Why necessary:

Abdominal muscles are stretched and weakened by the hormonal influences of pregnancy and altered posture during pregnancy. This could lead to pelvic instability, muscle imbalance, long-term back problems, lack of support, poor figure and loss of self-esteem.

Transversus

It is inadvisable to kneel on all fours until after all bleeding has stopped (approximately 4–6 weeks) because of the remote possibility of an air embolus entering the raw placental site.

Starting position – side-lying or crook-lying:

Lying on one side with both knees bent up and a pillow between the legs or lying on the back with knees bent up and feet flat on the bed.

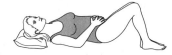

Figure 10.12 Starting position: crook-lying.

The exercise

• Keeping the spine in the mid position, breathe in and whilst breathing out, gently draw in the lower abdominal muscles towards the spine. Hold this position for up to 10 seconds, continuing to breathe normally, then relax slowly. Repeat up to 10 times.

Starting position – sitting:

Sitting well back on a dining-type chair with the feet on the floor. Place hands on the abdomen below the umbilicus with the fingers towards midline.

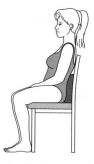

Figure 10.13 Starting position: sitting.

The exercise

• Keeping the spine in the mid position, breathe in and whilst breathing out, gently draw in the lower abdominal muscles away from the fingers towards the spine. Hold this position for up to 10 seconds, continuing to breathe normally, then relax slowly. Repeat up to 10 times.

Starting position – standing:

Standing with the weight evenly on both feet.

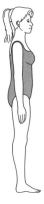

Figure 10.14 Starting position: standing.

The exercise

• Keeping the spine in the mid position, breathe in and whilst breathing out, gently draw in the lower abdominal muscles towards the spine. Hold this position for up to 10 seconds, continuing to breathe normally, then relax slowly. Repeat up to 10 times.

Frequency:

Several times a day in any of the different positions. Can be done whilst feeding, bathing baby, changing nappies. Transversus and the pelvic floor should be co-activated before performing activities such as changing position, climbing stairs, moving and handling objects. When standing for any length of time always tighten transversus and the pelvic floor muscles gently.

Pelvic tilting

Starting position – crook-lying:

Lying with the knees bent up and the feet flat on the bed or the floor.

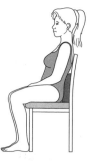

Figure 10.15 Starting position: crook-lying.

The exercise

- Pull in the abdominal muscles, tighten the buttock muscles and press the small of the back down onto the support. Hold for a count of 5, breathing normally, then relax. Repeat up to 10 times. This can also be done more rhythmically to ease tension in the back whenever necessary.

Starting position – supported sitting:

Sitting well back on a dining-type chair.

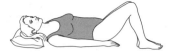

Figure 10.16 Starting position: supported sitting.

The exercise

- Pull in the abdominals, tighten the buttock muscles and press the small of the back into the back of the chair. Hold for a count of 5, breathing normally, then relax. Repeat up to 10 times.

Starting position – reverse sitting:

Sitting the opposite way round on a chair with the arms round the back of the chair.

The exercise

- Pull in the abdominals, tighten the buttock muscles, slightly rounding the lower back, and hold for a count of 5, breathing normally, then relax. Repeat up to 10 times.

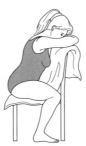

Figure 10.17   Starting position: reverse sitting.

Starting position – standing:

Standing tall with feet slightly apart.

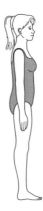

Figure 10.18   Starting position: standing.

The exercise

- Pull in the abdominal muscles and tuck in the buttocks. Hold for a count of 5, breathing normally, then relax. Repeat 10 times.

Frequency:

Several times a day in the different positions to relieve backache.

Advice:

- brace transversus and the pelvic floor before performing any functional activities
- brace transversus and the pelvic floor when standing

- the pelvic tilting exercise can also be performed rhythmically (rocking) to relieve backache
- correct standing posture using mirror
- always distribute weight evenly
- refer to an women's health physiotherapist if there are persistent back problems.

Core trunk stability exercises

To encourage transversus to stabilize the pelvis while movements of the lower limb are performed, the following exercises may be introduced about 5–10 days after a normal delivery if there are no musculoskeletal pelvic problems.

Starting position:

Sitting with feet flat on the floor and hands over the lower abdominal muscles.

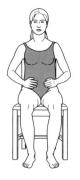

Figure 10.19 Starting position: sitting.

The exercise

- Draw in the transversus and pelvic floor muscles and raise one knee so the foot is a couple of inches off the floor. Hold for up to five seconds making sure the pelvis and spine remain level. Repeat five times with each leg. Gradually increase the hold to 10 seconds and repeat 10 times.

Frequency:

Two to three times a day.

Starting position:

Side-lying with both knees bent up in front.

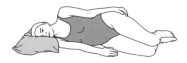

Figure 10.20   Starting position: side-lying.

The exercise

- Draw in transversus and the pelvic floor and lift the top knee by turning the hip outwards whilst keeping the heels together. Hold for up to five seconds making sure the pelvis or spine do not rotate. Repeat five times with each leg. Gradually increase the hold to 10 seconds and repeat 10 times.

Frequency:

Two to three times a day.

Starting position:

Side-lying with the underneath knee bent backwards.

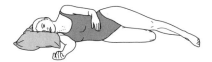

Figure 10.21   Starting position: side-lying.

The exercise

- Draw in the lower abdomen and raise the top leg up towards the ceiling keeping it in line with the body. Hold for up to five seconds making sure the back and pelvis do not rotate. Repeat five times with each leg. Gradually increase the hold to 10 seconds and repeat 10 times. Over the next few weeks progress to controlling the pelvis and spine whilst lifting the leg towards the ceiling with the hip rotated outwards.

Frequency:

Two to three times a day.

Starting position:

Crook-lying with knees bent up and feet flat on the floor, hands over the lower abdominal muscles.

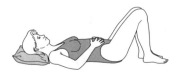

Figure 10.22   Starting position: crook-lying.

The exercise

- Pull in the lower abdomen and let the right knee lower outwards slightly controlling it to make sure that the pelvis stays level and the back stays flat. Slowly return the knee to the upright position. Repeat five times with alternate knees. Gradually increase repetitions up to 10. Over the next few weeks, progress to controlling the pelvis as the knee is lowered further.

Frequency:

Two to three times a day.

Starting position:

Crook-lying with knees bent up and feet flat on the floor, hands over the lower abdomen.

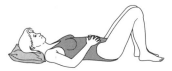

Figure 10.23   Starting position: crook-lying.

The exercise

- Pull in the lower abdomen and gently slide the heel of one leg downwards keeping the back flat and the pelvis level. Stop if the pelvis starts to move. Slowly return the knee to the bent position. Repeat five times with alternate legs. Gradually increase repetitions up to 10. Over the next few weeks, progress to controlling the pelvis whilst straightening the leg further.

EVALUATION OF TEACHING

It is now time for the educator to evaluate her performance as a teacher of these basic physical skills. Did the feedback indicate that all the relevant teaching points had been included? Does the reader feel more confident? Is further practice needed before introducing these skills to groups of antenatal or postnatal women? When the educator has mastered the teaching of the basic exercises, she may like to include the following additional exercises in her preparation for parenthood programme. These are chosen for the pregnant woman and are not appropriate postnatally.

ADDITIONAL ANTENATAL EXERCISES

Shoulder, arm and chest exercises

Aim of exercises:

To tone the shoulder and pectoral muscles and relieve upper backache and pressure in the shoulder region and upper ribs.

Why necessary:

Kyphosis often occurs in pregnancy and may cause aching on shoulders and upper back. Rib flare causes pressure under the ribs. Oedema causes pressure, which could lead to tingling in fingers and in the shoulder region. Breasts increase in size and weight and require increased support.

Starting position:

Sitting on chair with back well supported or tailor-sitting

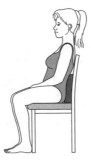

Figure 10.24 Starting position: sitting.

The exercises

- Raise and lower both shoulders together slowly. Repeat 5–10 times.

- Rest fingers on shoulders. Slowly and rhythmically bring both elbows forwards, upwards, backwards and then down, making large backward circles with the elbows. Repeat 5–10 times.
- Slowly stretch the right arm above the head and lower. Do the same with the left arm. Repeat 5–10 times. An added lift is gained if the trunk is bent very slightly to the opposite side while stretching.
- Lift elbows to shoulder height. Make a loose fist with one hand and clasp the other round it. Slowly press hands together and release. Repeat this exercise 5–10 times. Change hands and repeat.

Frequency:

Once/twice per day.

Advice:

- breathe easily during exercises
- do not arch the lower back during these exercises
- be aware of posture of upper back and so avoid slumping (slouching) forwards.

Stretching exercises

Aim of exercises:

To prepare women physically and psychologically for taking up and holding wide advantageous positions for labour and delivery.

Why necessary:

There is shortness and tightness of the muscles of the calves and inner thighs, and ligaments of the groin, hips and lower limbs.

Warning: Stretching exercises should always be preceded by warm-up exercises, and pregnant women must never overstretch.

Starting position:

Standing at arm's length from a wall with palms pressed against it, one foot behind the other.

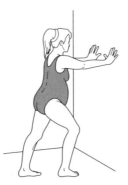

Figure 10.25 Starting position: standing with one foot behind the other.

The exercise

- Lean gently into the wall, bending the front leg and both elbows slightly. A stretch in the calf muscle will be felt in the back leg. Hold the stretch for half to one minute. Change legs and repeat. If this feels very easy, move the back leg further away from the other leg.

Frequency:

Once/twice per day.

Starting position:

Squatting, holding on to a firm support or partner.

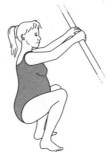

Figure 10.26 Starting position: squatting.

The exercise

- Practise holding this position for half a minute and gradually increase to one minute.

Frequency:

Once/twice per day.

Starting Position:

Sitting on the floor with the back supported and the soles of the feet together, knees resting on a pillow.

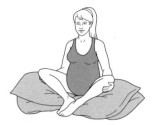

Figure 10.27   Starting position: sitting on floor with back supported.

The exercise

• Keep the feet as close to the pelvis as possible and bold the position for as long as you are comfortable.

Frequency:

Once/twice per day.

Starting position:

Sitting on the floor with the back supported and the soles of the feet together, hands holding ankles and feet pulled in towards the perineum.

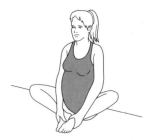

Figure 10.28   Starting position: sitting on floor with back supported.

The exercise

• Allow the weight of the legs to take the knees down towards the floor for half a minute and gradually increase to one minute.

Frequency:

Once/twice per day.

Starting position:

Sitting with the back supported and the legs out in front and wide apart, keeping the knees straight.

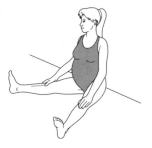
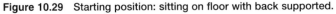

Figure 10.29 Starting position: sitting on floor with back supported.

The exercise

• Pull the feet up towards the body at the ankle, without bending the knees. Hold the stretch for half a minute increasing to one minute.

Frequency:

Once/twice per day.

Advice:

• remember to warm up the body before starting stretches
• always repeat stretches slowly
• at first a point will be reached where the stretch is felt; breathe easily until the sensation ceases staying with the stretch
• the range of movement will gradually be increased and the body will feel more flexible and relaxed
• never force movements
• the squatting position may only be able to be held with heels off the ground at first
• follow stretching with a warm bath or shower.

WARNING

These stretching exercises should not be practised if any pain is experienced in the symphysis pubis area as this might indicate separation at the joint (see Ch. 3). Caution should also be taken if there is any backache and exercises should be stopped if any pain is felt. Stretches should never be developed (forced) during pregnancy because of the laxity of ligaments (see Ch. 2).

FURTHER ADVICE

It is always better to advise women to exercise for a short period regularly, rather than for longer, less frequent sessions. They should not exercise when feeling tired or unwell, and should build up gradually after a break from exercising. Individuals will progress at different rates, depending on pre-pregnancy fitness, age, delivery and parity and should exercise to suit their personal needs and comfort.

11

Programme planning for physical skills

The antenatal team   143
Physical skills content of antenatal
  and postnatal classes   144
  Early pregnancy (earlybird)   144
  Women only   145
  Couples   146
  Caesarean delivery   147
  Transcutaneous electrical nerve
    stimulation (TENS)   147
  Ethnic minorities   148

Teenagers' clubs   148
Refreshers   149
Ward classes   149
Individuals   149
Postnatal classes   149
Community postnatal
  classes   150
Postnatal reunion   150
References   150
Further Reading   151

This chapter makes suggestions as to types of classes where physical skills are appropriate, and outlines the content of these skills for each type of class. It will not discuss parentcraft topics.

THE ANTENATAL TEAM

The composition of the antenatal education team will vary in different centres. Ideally it consists of a midwife, a women's health physiotherapist and a health visitor. An obstetrician, anaesthetist, National Childbirth Trust (NCT) teacher, dietician and social worker may be involved for occasional talks during the series. Outside speakers may also be invited to special meetings to discuss such subjects as car safety seats, toys and feeding. Parents who have recently given birth may be invited to share their experiences.

A women's health physiotherapist is the professional with the knowledge and expertise to teach the physical/practical skills input to antenatal groups (see Tripartite Agreement p ix, x). Physiotherapists specialising in obstetrics are in short supply and, if one is not available, the midwife or health visitor may be required to teach exercises, relaxation and coping strategies for labour.

There can be no fixed standard scheme of antenatal education. Choice of type of classes, content, length, time, numbers, leaders and venue will all depend on local, economic, and social factors and will vary considerably from place to place. Discussion with the women and their partners should always take place at the start of any programme to ascertain what the group would like included in the course. They always request breathing and relaxation with a view to coping with labour, and often ask how to relieve discomforts in pregnancy.

Health and safety precautions should always be considered when choosing both venue and optimum numbers for an antenatal group that will be performing exercises and relaxation. Classes that are too large do not allow the teacher to supervise individually or observe women who may be looking uncomfortable, nor do they allow space for exercises or relaxation to be practised effectively. It is suggested that eight to 12 in a group works well and allows for the fostering of close personal relationships, which can add to the client's satisfaction (Wilson, 1990). It would be ideal for two members of the antenatal team to lead a two-hour session together, but this may not be economically possible. If just one professional is with the group at any one time, another person should be nearby in case of emergency.

Security is important in community settings, particularly at night, and this aspect may influence the choice of venue for an evening course.

PHYSICAL SKILLS CONTENT OF ANTENATAL AND POSTNATAL CLASSES

Early pregnancy (earlybird)

The hormonal effects on the musculoskeletal system occur very early in pregnancy (see Ch. 2), so it makes sense to encourage couples to attend early pregnancy classes, for example, at about 12 weeks. Combes & Schonveld (1992) suggested that it is most appropriate to cover health and lifestyle issues in the first three months of pregnancy when they are most significant for the health of the mother and baby. However, in practice the woman is often extremely tired at this stage and may still be feeling nauseous. Her partner may only just be coming to terms with the fact that he is to become a father. These factors often mean that attendances at this time are low. Inviting couples to evening sessions a little later, for example, at about 16 weeks, usually results in a better attendance. Unfortunately, resources often limit this early session to a one-off, whereas two or three sessions would allow time for information to be assimilated at a reasonable pace and give the parents-to-be the opportunity to ask questions.

If there is only one evening allocated, then the desirable physical skills input would be a discussion and demonstration/practice of comfortable postures in all positions, both resting and working, correct moving and lifting techniques, transversus, pelvic-floor and circulatory exercises. If the numbers are large, the exercises may have to be performed on chairs, but it should always be possible to demonstrate other positions. Advice on sufficient rest and delegation of chores should be included and if a second evening is available, relaxation would be the obvious addition. It is very much easier to learn the transversus and pelvic-floor exercises at this stage of pregnancy than later. Prevention of backache and postural problems is very much better than cure (Mantle et al 1981).

Sometimes these early-pregnancy evenings are more popular in local clinics so that couples do not have to travel to a central hospital. However there may be issues around security.

Women only

These classes usually take place during the daytime from about 30–32 weeks of pregnancy when many women have finished work. A two-hour session allows time for practising physical skills, comfort breaks and refreshments, parentcraft discussions, demonstrations and/or visits. Classes often lead to friendships and local support groups which last throughout early parenthood.

A preparation for parenthood course commonly consists of four to six two-hour sessions. At the first session, it must be established whether anyone has any physical problems, for example, long-term back pain, asthma, which could possibly be exacerbated by different positions. These women must always understand that they are free to omit any position or activity with which they are not comfortable, or to try an alternative.

During the first session, discussing the musculoskeletal and circulatory changes occurring during pregnancy will lead on to the need for good backcare and exercises to prevent long-term problems in the future. Foot and leg exercises, specific abdominal exercises and discussion and experimentation with comfortable and practical postures for daily activities could all be included in this session. The group will volunteer positions and situations of stress when this topic is discussed and a chosen technique of relaxation can be introduced. Many physiotherapists and midwives prefer the physiological relaxation described in Chapter 5, but if a woman has her own method of relaxation, she could continue using it. Breathing awareness is a logical accompaniment to relaxation. The group can discuss opportunities for the practice of relaxation. It is not good use of the professional's time to let the group spend too long relaxing during the class unless it is a convenient time for her to go and make the tea! However the women should need no encouraging to practise the relaxation technique at home. Relaxation in different positions, good postures and correct lifting techniques should be practised in every session.

It may be better to introduce the topic of the pelvic floor in the second session rather than in the first, as sufficient time is needed to emphasise its importance and to practise the exercise. Members of the group can suggest memory-links and suitable times and situations to practise at home and at work.

The next two or three sessions will cover labour and could include positions of ease for first stage, relaxation, breathing awareness and adaptations when necessary (see Ch. 6), massage, pain relief (including a demonstration and practice with TENS), practical positions for second stage, alternative positions for delivery and the role of the partner. Ideally, these sessions will link in with topics previously covered in the parentcraft programme. The women appreciate at least one evening session during the course to which they can bring their partners to rehearse labour, visit the delivery suite, neonatal unit and postnatal wards, and maybe watch a relevant video.

As women are staying increasingly shorter times after delivery, it is important to stress the 'do's and don'ts' for the immediate postnatal period (see Ch. 9). The postnatal scene could be considered in the last session. Postnatal exercises, the need for adequate rest and relaxation, posture, lifting, resuming normal and sporting activities are all topics which could be discussed at this time. The group should be taught how to check for diastasis recti postnatally. They should be told that, if they are worried, they should seek the advice of their women's health physiotherapist or midwife. Core stability exercises can be demonstrated to the group at this last session and an illustrated postnatal programme given out as a reminder.

Women are now working longer into their pregnancies and if in full-time employment may find evening classes each week exhausting. An alternative is to provide weekend classes, which only necessitate one or two days' attendance, for example, two Saturdays one or two weeks apart. A whole weekend would be too exhausting for full-time workers. It is not possible for all would-be participants (male or female) to be able to access daytime classes for work commitments may involve travel away from home during the week.

Couples

It must be remembered that couples are not always of the opposite sex. The birthing partner may be another female of the woman's choice, for example, sister, friend, or the woman may be in an all-female relationship. In many areas the demand for couples' classes has increased so dramatically over the last few years that mornings/afternoons for women only are relatively few. Even though many men are allowed time off by liberated employers for antenatal classes, the preference for evening or weekend sessions far outweighs that for daytime classes. It was found that half the men attending just one evening session with their partners did not find it very enjoyable (Hassey 1990). They wanted to be able to attend all the classes with their partners as the one class did not give sufficient time.

When a whole series of couples' classes is offered, the partners enjoy joining in the exercises and relaxation and should be encouraged to do so, rather than watching. If space is at a premium, they may have to perform the exercises in alternative positions. The couples can practise relaxation and coping strategies for labour in pairs and, where wedges and pillows are in short supply, the men can act as backrests and supports for different positions. Practical massage sessions are both fun and beneficial. The birthing partners will learn a skill with which they can help the women both during pregnancy and labour. The role of the supporter in labour can be discussed as can worries expressed by both partners. Often, the couples gain from separating for part of the evening to allow different topics to be discussed by the partners or women separately.

Caesarean delivery

In areas with a high rate of caesarean deliveries it is worth considering devoting classes solely to mothers who will be having an elective caesarean birth. In a survey held to evaluate consumer satisfaction of antenatal classes, only 18% of those who had undergone a caesarean delivery were satisfied with the antenatal preparation they received (Hassey, 1990).

These women and their partners will not be as interested in adaptations of breathing for late first and second stage, but will want to know the pros and cons of epidural versus general anaesthesia and more about the actual procedure. The mothers will need to learn how to move up and down and in and out of bed after delivery (see Ch. 9), without increasing pain. Circulatory exercises immediately following pelvic surgery are extremely important, especially after epidural or spinal anaesthesia, as there will be increased fluid and the leg muscles may feel lethargic. Positions for coughing, feeding and other activities with the baby can be demonstrated and practised.

Partners and relatives may need reminding that a caesarean delivery is not the easy way out. Instead, they have to appreciate that the mother has undergone major surgery in addition to giving birth and that she will take longer to recuperate than a woman who has had a vaginal delivery. Practical advice about resuming activities such as driving and housework may be discussed now, so the couple can plan for extra help if this is possible (see Ch. 9).

Transcutaneous electrical nerve stimulation (TENS)

If the demand is sufficient, it is appropriate to arrange a special time for couples who are interested in using TENS in labour (see Ch. 7). Women should experience its effects before deciding that they would like to use it in labour as occasionally a woman finds she does not find the sensation comfortable. A video illustrating the way the obstetric TENS works will save technical explanations and could be borrowed by interested couples if there is insufficient time to show it to a group. Different models can be demonstrated and the advantages discussed before the couple decide whether or not to hire one (see Ch. 7). Some delivery suites have sufficient TENS units to be able to lend one to a couple before the birth, or have a rental scheme in operation. However, many couples choose to hire their own. Partners should be taught when, where and how to site the electrodes and supervised doing this if possible.

Ethnic minorities

In some areas with high ethnic minority populations, it may be desirable to hold special classes for these women. An interpreter or link worker can be employed, but it may not be possible to translate directly as certain English phrases and explanations are unacceptable to other cultures. Alternative descriptions need to be discussed with a professional who could help with this. The extended family is much more widespread in some of these communities and it may be necessary to gain the confidence and encouragement of the female head of the family before inviting the women to attend classes. Handouts cannot be directly translated into other languages because of the different acceptable terminology and professional advice must be sought before preparing leaflets for ethnic minorities. Another problem is the number of dialects that exist in any one language, making it impossible to include all of them. Many women are not encouraged to participate fully in everyday activities, and some may not be able to read. If an interpreter is used, it should always be a female, as some of these women are not willing to discuss anything related to sex – even pelvic-floor exercises – with a male. Occasionally, it may be appropriate for a midwife or health visitor to hold a group session in the home of one of the group members.

Teenagers' clubs

Teenagers' clubs or groups fulfil a very real need as long as they provide a relaxed atmosphere where the girls feel they can do their own thing with no pressure to conform. Organisers should not be discouraged if the girls do not attend regularly, but just drop in when they feel like it. A companion of either sex should be invited to accompany the teenager. A loosely structured programme is all that is possible (Evans & Parker 1985; Will 1990), and it has been found that the teenagers are very reluctant to join in any exercises at all, though relaxation has slightly more appeal. Hopefully, demonstrations of positions and coping strategies for labour will be recalled when needed, even though they have not been practised.

Refreshers

Refresher classes for multiparous women may include physical skills only, if the mothers feel they are happy about baby care. Sessions can be held for one or two hours as a one-off or as a series over three to four weeks, and can cover anything the mothers request. Usually they ask for relaxation and breathing. Sometimes the mothers have delivered at home or in other units and welcome the opportunity for a visit to the delivery suite where they are booked to have this baby. Mothers who have longer gaps between pregnancies and no ties with toddlers often prefer to attend a full course with first-time mothers. They may have either forgotten parentcraft techniques, or need updating as newer ideas have emerged since their last delivery. These women can be a valuable addition to the classes especially in discussion on postnatal activities.

Ward classes

When women have been admitted to the antenatal ward or day unit during their pregnancy, they have plenty of time to discuss parentcraft topics and learn such physical skills as are safe to practise, even if bed rest has been advised. Relaxation will always be beneficial and a good time to hold a group session would be just before the afternoon rest period. If the woman is confined to bed, foot and leg exercises are essential to prevent circulatory stasis, particularly if there is oedema present due to hypertension. If the woman is able to join the regular antenatal class, she will enjoy the change from the ward atmosphere as well as learning new skills.

Individuals

Some women will prefer not to attend classes for social or economic reasons, but antenatal preparation can be given on a one-to-one basis in clinic or at home by the midwife. Any woman with special needs because of a permanent or temporary disability should be referred to a women's health physiotherapist if at all possible. She will require individual assessment and, depending on her needs, adaptations of supports, starting positions or exercises may allow the woman to join in the regular antenatal sessions. It maybe more appropriate, however, for advice and instruction to be continued on an individual basis in the local clinic or the woman's own home.

Postnatal classes

In these days of early discharges and demand-feeding, it is practically impossible to arrange group postnatal classes in hospital. This is a pity as they can be fun and motivate the mothers to practise their exercises.

Ideally, all women should receive individual postnatal exercise instruction and advice before leaving hospital. With current restraints, however, this is not always possible and the onus is falling increasingly on the midwife to provide this service when the woman has been transferred home (see Ch. 10).

Community postnatal classes

Some authorities run postnatal exercise classes in the community along similar lines to antenatal classes. Mothers can attend at weekly intervals for as long as they wish and babies are invited too! Abdominal muscles are assessed and the core stability exercises are progressed, preparing mothers to return to more strenuous sporting activities.

Postnatal reunion

The provision of a monthly reunion class allows a group of mothers and their babies to meet up with each other and the antenatal teachers approximately six weeks after the last mother in the group was due to deliver. It is a forum for general exchange of notes and ideas, where any physical problems or anxieties can be brought up. This is a good time to check that the women are not suffering from any backache, urinary or faecal problems. The abdominals should be checked to ensure there is no diastasis of the rectus muscles and that the transversus exercise is being performed correctly. If any problems are present the mother should be referred on to a women's health physiotherapist. It might also be at this time that the woman is aware of dyspareunia, which may also be treated by a women's health physiotherapist (see Ch. 8). The reunion may be purely a social and problem-airing session or could include a revision of postnatal exercises, baby-massage and suggestions for future activities. The postnatal reunion is also an ideal opportunity for the evaluation of the preparation for parenthood sessions attended by the group. Combes & Schonveld (1992) stated that more attention could be given to the provision of support groups during the first six weeks, and after the first four or five months postnatally.

REFERENCES

Combes G, Schonveld A 1992 Life will never be the same again. Health Education Authority, London
Evans G, Parker P 1985 Preparing teenagers for parenthood. Midwives Chronicle vol 98, 1172:239–240
Hassey L 1990 An evaluation of antenatal classes. Journal of The Association of Chartered Physiotherapists in Obstetrics and Gynaecology 67:17–18

Mantle M J, Holmes J, Currey J L F 1981 Backache in pregnancy 11: Prophylactic Influence of Back Care Classes. Rheumatalogical Rehabilitation 20:227–232

Will A 1990 A physiotherapist's view of teenage antenatal classes. Journal of The Association of Chartered Physiotherapists in Obstetrics and Gynaecology 67:15–16

Wilson P 1990 Antenatal Teaching. Faber & Faber, London

FURTHER READING

Campion M J 1990 The Baby Challenge: a handbook on pregnancy for women with a physical disability. Routledge, London

Rooke J 1991 Cultural differences in pregnancy. Journal of The Association of Chartered Physiotherapists in Obstetrics and Gynaecology 69:7–8

Schott J, Priest J 2002 Leading Antenatal Classes. A Practical Guide. Books for Midwives Press, Oxford

12

Alternative approaches to fitness antenatally and postpartum

Aerobic exercise 158
  Antenatal session 158
  Postnatal session 159
  Facilities and equipment 159
  Clothing 160
Aquanatal exercise 160
  Benefits of aquanatal exercise 160
  Contra-indications to aquanatal
    exercise 161
  Facilities 162
  Equipment 163
  Staffing 163
  Clothing 164

Antenatal 164
Postnatal 164
Points to remember when
  teaching aquanatal exercise 165
Safeguards for the
  professionals 165
Pilates 166
Summary of advice for exercise
  teachers 167
Summary of advice for women 168
References 168
Further reading 170
Videos 170

The exercise content of preparation for parenthood programmes (see Ch. 4) is generally limited to specific abdominal and pelvic floor exercises and many women request guidance on further beneficial exercise. It has been noted that nearly 45% of women of childbearing age exercise (Sady & Carpenter 1989) and, when pregnant, many of these wish to continue. Zhang & Savitz (1996) found that 42% of nearly 1000 exercising women surveyed did continue to exercise during pregnancy. Women who do not normally exercise often become more health-conscious in pregnancy and decide to start an exercise programme to improve their health and fitness (Hammer et al 2000) and want to know what exercise to do, whether sport can be continued, and what should be avoided.

The physiology and benefits of exercise in general are well known and are summarized in Boxes 12.1 and 12.2. Just as in non-pregnant exercisers, there are also beneficial physical and psychological effects for the pregnant woman (Box 12.3).

Cardiovascular fitness is maintained (Kramer 2002), weight gain and fat retention are limited (Clapp 2000). It has been found that women who continued to exercise during pregnancy had a lower incidence of abdominal and vaginal operative delivery, a shorter active labour in those who were delivered vaginally, a quicker recovery after birth and improved physical fitness (Clapp 2000). Yeo et al (2000) studied women who were at risk of maternal hypertension during pregnancy and postulated that exercise may lower the diastolic blood pressure, whilst Hartmann & Bung (1999)

Box 12.1 Physiology of exercise:

- initial rise in BP followed by drop in BP
- increased cardiac output
- increased heart rate
- increased respiratory rate
- increased rate of perceived exertion (RPE)
- increased temperature
- increased skin colour
- possible sweating, palpitations, aching muscles, fatigue, pain, nausea if too much exercise.

Box 12.2 General beneficial effects of exercise:

- improved circulation and cardiovascular fitness
- improved breathing awareness and control
- improved postural awareness
- strengthens specific muscle groups
- increases endurance and stamina
- reduces fatigue, improves sleep
- enhances psychological well-being
- reduces stress and anxiety
- encourages social interaction.

Box 12.3 Potential additional benefits of exercise for pregnant woman:

- maintains/improves cardiovascular fitness
- limits weight gain and fat retention
- improves attitudes and mental state
- reduces anxiety and insomnia
- easier and less complicated labour
- assists a speedier postnatal recovery
- may lower diastolic BP
- may prevent gestational diabetes
- may reduce risk of LSCS in nulliparous women.

---

proposed that exercise may prevent gestational diabetes. It has been shown statistically that there was a higher level of psychological well-being, improved body image and lower physical discomfort amongst pregnant women who exercised regularly compared with those who did not exercise. These women also displayed less anxiety and suffered less from insomnia (Goodwin et al 2000).

Box 12.4   Potential benefits of exercise to the fetus:

- reduced growth of fat organ
- increased stress tolerance
- advanced neurobehavioural maturation
- fewer signs of stress during delivery
- high Apgar scores at delivery
- enhanced fetoplacental growth
- may reduce risk of LSCS in nulliparous women.

Some studies reported benefits to the fetus when the mother exercised (Box 12.4). Clapp (2000) claimed there was reduced growth of the fat organ, increased stress tolerance and evidence of advanced neurobehavioural maturation at five years of age. Clapp et al (2000) maintained that exercise during pregnancy enhanced fetoplacental growth and Henriksson-Larsen (1999) found that babies of exercising mothers showed less signs of stress during delivery and had higher Apgar scores after delivery than those born to non-exercising mothers. MacPhail et al (2000) claimed a possible reduced risk of caesarean delivery in nulliparous exercising women.

However, changes take place in the body during pregnancy that can affect exercise performance and these should be taken into consideration when giving advice on exercise or planning exercise programmes. The heart rate and stroke volume are already increased (Bush 1992) and will increase by approximately a further 15% during exercise (Wallace & Wiswell 1991). The respiratory centre is more sensitive to carbon dioxide so the woman may become increasingly breathless. There is an increase in weight and the effect of relaxin has made ligaments more pliable, leading to joints becoming less stable. As the uterus becomes larger, there is an alteration in lumbar lordosis and the pelvis is tilted forwards, altering the centre of gravity. The woman can lose her balance more easily and is less nimble (see Ch. 2). These factors could lead to the woman being more prone to musculoskeletal injury when exercising, although Jones (2000) concludes that there is no real evidence to support this being a problem.

It is advised that women should avoid hyperthermia throughout pregnancy since it could be injurious to the fetus (Artal & Buckenmeyer 1995). During the first trimester, raised maternal core temperatures may bring about teratogenic effects. It is suggested by Polden and Mantle (1990) that intensive exercise during pregnancy might result in intrauterine growth retardation, preterm labour and, due to redistribution of blood flow, fetal distress. However more recent evidence does not support this as studies found that any rises in core temperature after moderate exercise were well within the safety limits of below 38.5°C (Clapp 2000, O'Neill 1996), and Brenner et al (1999) found that a maternal heart rate of up to 170 beats per minute did not induce fetal distress. Riemann & Kanstrup Hansen (2000) reported higher birth weights from women who exercised three or four times weekly compared with those who exercised less or more than that frequency. Postulated dangers of exercise in pregnancy are summarized in Box 12.5.

Box 12.5 Postulated dangers of exercise in pregnancy:

- reduction in blood flow to uterus
- breathlessness
- risk of maternal injury
- risk of maternal and fetal hypoglycaemia
- hyperthermia
- fatigue
- intrauterine growth retardation (IUGR), premature labour – after intensive exercise.

What advice should be given to women and what can be offered to them? Provided that there is no obstetric problem or pre-existing disease, moderate exercise is safe and women should be encouraged to maintain their prepregnancy activity level (Clapp 2000). However, women should not take up anything new which is strenuous during pregnancy and a modest reduction of the training programme would be wise during the last trimester. The types of exercise that provide the best cardiovascular and psychological benefits during pregnancy include walking, cycling and swimming.

Sady & Carpenter (1989) described a moderate aerobic programme lasting 30 minutes, three days per week with the heart rate not exceeding 150 beats per minute. Artal & Buckenmeyer (1995) suggested an intensity range of 'somewhat hard' on the Borg rating of perceived exertion (RPE). Some exercise, for example, high-impact aerobics, and any contact sport or physical activities involving sudden starts and changes of direction, for example, tennis or squash, are contraindicated during pregnancy. Any sport where there is risk of an abdominal blow or breast trauma should be avoided and downhill skiing or water skiing should be discouraged in later pregnancy. Scuba-diving should be avoided due to the risk of decompression sickness in the fetus (ACOG 2002). Women who normally horse-ride need to be warned about the risk of a fall and possible stress to the sacroiliac joint and spine. A gentle hack is safer and more sensible than more strenuous activities. Step classes are inadvisable because of the pressure on the symphysis pubis and the risk of musculoskeletal injury from a trip. With all types of sport and exercise, competition is generally inadvisable during pregnancy because of the anxiety and maximal efforts imposed (Revelli et al 1992).

Because of the demand for exercise in pregnancy and the postnatal period, specially designed aerobic exercise classes and aquanatal classes have been made available. Care must be taken to direct pregnant women only to those antenatal/postnatal aerobic and aquanatal exercise classes that are taken by qualified teachers who have undertaken a course relating to pregnancy and postpartum. They can provide expert advice and specially selected exercises for pregnancy and the postnatal period. Classes are suitable for women, whether they are used to exercise or not, because they are low-impact and not over-exerting and are tailored to the individual's needs. They will increase body-awareness and maintain mobility, tone and fitness levels. These sessions offer group support and extra care is taken of the woman. Antenatally they should supplement rather than replace preparation for parenthood classes.

Box 12.6 Contraindications to exercise in pregnancy:

- cardiovascular, respiratory or renal disease
- hypertension
- poorly controlled diabetes mellitus
- thyroid disease
- placenta praevia, history of bleeding
- raised temperature, fever
- history of risk of miscarriage, cervical incompetence
- history of premature labour
- multiple pregnancy
- intrauterine growthg retardation (IUGR).

Safety is of paramount importance and it is vital to screen each woman before she starts exercising (Ashton 1992). The contraindications to exercise in pregnancy (see Box 12.6) include such disorders of pregnancy as:

- threatened miscarriage
- preterm labour
- uterine haemorrhage
- placenta praevia
- pre-eclampsia
- intrauterine growth retardation (ACOG 2002).

Exercise is also contraindicated for women suffering from significant valvular or ischaemic heart disease, type I diabetes mellitus, peripheral vascular disease, uncontrolled hypertension and thyroid disease (Ezmerli 2000). Physical work must also be especially limited in multiple pregnancy and in women with respiratory illness. Screening should also include checking for musculoskeletal problems, for example, diastasis symphysis pubis, sacroiliac strain, back pain and continence problems.

Every exercising woman should stop exercising immediately and consult her doctor if one of the following symptoms appears: vaginal bleeding, abdominal pain, severe tachycardia, chest pain, severe breathlessness, headache, loss of muscle control, dizziness, calf pain/swelling, decreased fetal movements, ruptured membranes (ACOG 2002).

AEROBIC EXERCISE

Antenatal session

An antenatal exercise-to-music programme should begin with a warm-up session and short stretch. This can be followed by a gentle/moderate aerobic section designed to suit the woman's needs, muscle strengthening, stretching, cool-down and relaxation. Some floor work would be included. It is suggested that the aerobic section lasts for no more than 30 minutes (Artal & Buckenmeyer 1995). There should be no bouncy, jerky movements, no full extension or flexion of joints, and no quick changes of direction because of the compromised balance mentioned earlier. Breath-holding must be discouraged to prevent rise in intra-abdominal pressure, and muscle work needs to be varied.

The women will need to alter their level of exercise according to their stage of pregnancy (see above). Any exercise (or relaxation) normally performed lying flat on the back should be executed in a modified position after the fourth month of pregnancy because of the risk of developing the supine hypotensive syndrome (see Ch. 2).

The exercises include those that are especially relevant for the pregnant woman: pelvic tilting, pelvic-floor and stretching. The aim and advantage of each should be explained with emphasis on good technique, poise and posture in all movements. Concepts of good back care are also introduced. Particular care will be taken by a qualified instructor to avoid the inclusion of exercises that could be harmful for the pregnant woman, for instance: wide deep squats, lumbar extension. An active cool-down is especially important for the pregnant woman because venous pooling might occur with abrupt cessation of activity and venous return may already be hampered by the growing uterus (Sady & Carpenter 1989). A session would last for approximately 45 minutes in total and finish with relaxation.

It is not wise to exercise directly after a meal. It could be suggested that the women eat a light carbohydrate-rich snack about one hour before the start of the session. Artal & Buckenmeyer (1995) advised plenty of liquid before, during and after exercise to help prevent hyperthermia and dehydration.

Postnatal session

Postnatally, the mothers usually return to aerobic sessions from about six weeks following delivery. It is advised that, on average, mothers who have not exercised before pregnancy join the postnatal group at nine weeks post delivery (Ashton 1992). Benefits include improved cardiovascular fitness, significantly less weight retention and increased psychological well-being. Studies on postnatal women who were taking part in regular moderate exercise have not found any adverse effects on lactation (Dewey 1998; Fly et al 1998; McCrory et al 1999; Sampselle et al 1999). However it would be more comfortable if women exercised after feeding.

Consideration must be given to the physical changes that took place during pregnancy, remembering that joints are still vulnerable and the pelvic floor and abdominal muscles may still be weak (see Ch. 7). Screening is again essential and should include checking to ascertain if there are any pelvic floor (continence), back or symphysis pubis problems and women referred to a women's health physiotherapist if necessary. The abdomen should be palpated for possible diastasis of the rectus abdominis muscles before proceeding to abdominal work (see Chs. 8 and 9).

The programme for the postnatal session can be similar to that run antenatally. Exercise is adapted to suit the mother's individual needs and ability. The class can last up to an hour and may include a little more aerobic work and more strengthening exercises especially of the pelvic-floor and abdominal muscles. Again there is emphasis on good posture and back care. Finishing with relaxation is particularly relevant for this group.

Facilities and equipment

Ideally the venue should be close to adequate car parking so the woman is not struggling to carry baby in a car seat for any distance. A large, well-ventilated room is required with a non-slip floor surface, for example, wood or carpet. Cloakrooms with toilets should be nearby. A chair, at least two pillows and a small mat is required for each participant. Plenty of cold drinks must be available. If no music system is installed a portable cassette player can be used. Remember, batteries should be on hand in case there is no suitable source of electricity. Tapes for each type of exercise will be the personal choice of the teacher.

NB. Anyone using recorded music for classes in a public building must ensure they are covered by a PPL (Phonographic Performance Limited) licence for the premises, otherwise they will have to purchase one for their own use. There are strict copyright regulations that govern the playing of recorded music to a group.

Clothing

Good footwear is essential to provide adequate support to the feet and help avoid strains. A loose cotton shirt may be more comfortable antenatally than a tight leotard and all women need to wear a good supporting bra.

AQUANATAL EXERCISE

Aquanatal exercises are supervised group activities for the ante- or post-natal periods which take place in water. The exercise sessions are performed to music and can be executed in standing, lying, kneeling or squatting positions. It is not necessary to be able to swim to participate. There is a growing interest in these sessions and more and more women are requesting them.

Benefits of aquanatal exercise

Water is an excellent medium for the performance of exercise (see Box 12.7). It has beneficial effects on the musculoskeletal, respiratory and cardiovascular systems. McMurray et al (1990), found the plasma beta endorphin was significantly elevated when exercise took place in water during pregnancy. This may explain the psychological feeling of well-being of the pregnant woman following aquanatal sessions. The buoyancy of the water supports the weight of the body allowing easier movements with less strain on joints. The increased body weight and the change in the centre of gravity have a much smaller effect during a non-weight-bearing exercise (Revelli et al 1992). In a randomized study, Kihlstrand et al (1999) found

---

Box 12.7 Benefits of aquanatal exercise:

- plasma beta endorphins elevated
- body weight is supported – less strain on joints
- improved venous return
- reduction of lower limb oedema
- stimulates bowel function
- diuretic effect for up to four hours after session
- facilitates relaxation
- increases cardiovascular fitness
- increased tone in respiratory muscles
- a psychological effect appears to aid sleep.

that exercise in water significantly reduced the incidence of back pain in the second half of pregnancy. The hydrostatic pressure of the water increases venous return and the deeper the water the more beneficial the effect on the venous return. The pressure may help to reduce lower limb oedema (Kent et al 1999) and stimulate bowel function. The resistance of the water around the chest wall will help to improve respiratory function by increasing the work required by the respiratory muscles. This is particularly beneficial for women hoping to use the birthing pool. There is also a diuretic effect on women after 30–40 minutes in the water, which lasts until four hours after the session. If the temperature is adequate and floats are available, water is an excellent facilitator of relaxation. Hartmann & Bung (1999) highly recommended aquatic exercise during pregnancy provided potential dangers and contra-indications are observed.

Contra-indications to aquanatal exercise

The women participating in antenatal or postnatal aquanatal regimes should be carefully checked against the criteria in Box 12.8 which could be contra-indications to group therapy in water. Women with these conditions would not be included unless their problem is minor and they are monitored frequently. (This latter criterion might mean that extra members of staff would be needed).

Box 12.8 Contraindications to aquanatal exercise:

As for aerobic exercise plus:

- excessive fear of water
- skin lesions
- uncontrolled epilepsy
- respiratory insufficiency
- ruptured membranes in pregnancy
- bleeding postpartum
- unhealed perineum
- any infective condition
- IUGR
- Uncontrolled diabetes.

Women with specific pregnancy-related conditions including history of the following should also be discouraged from aquanatal sessions:

- history of spontaneous abortion
- shirodkar suture (cervical cerclage)
- pregnancy-induced hypertension
- ante-partum haemorrhage

- intrauterine growth retardation (IUGR)
- ruptured membranes
- history of premature labour.

If a problem has settled, for instance early bleeding in pregnancy, a letter from the consultant obstetrician stating that the woman is fit for aquanatal exercises would be required. Some obstetricians are happy to allow their women to participate with a shirodkar suture in situ, but permission must be sought. It is interesting to note that a study of Oxford women who were suffering from pregnancy hypertension found that their blood pressure, which was checked before, during and after an aquanatal session, was lower and stayed lower for up to four hours after the session than it had been before the start (Evans G personal communication 2002). If a woman presents with musculoskeletal problems, the midwife should consult with a women's health physiotherapist before the woman joins the group.

Specific postnatal contraindications

These would be:

- unhealed perineum
- vaginal discharge
- any infective condition.

Again, if a woman presents with any musculoskeletal problems, the midwife should consult with a women's health physiotherapist before the mother is included in the group.

Facilities

Ideally the sessions should take place in a swimming pool, which is closed to the general public and where the water temperature can be increased to at least 30°C for antenatal sessions, but lower than this would be satisfactory for postnatal classes. The surrounding air temperature should be the same as that of the water to prevent chilling. Cooler water is not conducive to relaxation, but if the water is too warm, it may lead to vasodilatation, hypotension, fainting and fatigue. If the woman's blood pressure is low to start with she should not be in a very warm pool. Hospital hydrotherapy pools may be too warm if higher than 36°C unless the temperature can be reduced, as the higher temperature may allow an increase in maternal core temperature, which can be harmful for the baby (Artal & Buckenmeyer 1995). An ideal depth would be to the level of the xiphisternum. If the depth of the water increases to above the level of the xiphisternum vertical balance may be threatened. However if there is insufficient depth, some movements could be performed kneeling or squatting in shallower water to allow the level to reach the optimum. Women should wear a bra in the water to support the breast tissue and should avoid jumping movements to prevent breast discomfort. Potential dangers are listed in Box 12.9.

Box 12.9 Potential dangers of aquanatal exercise in pregnancy:

- increase in core temperature
- increase in energy expenditure
- fatigue due to not recognizing amount of work done
- heat loss if water too shallow and too much inactivity.

There may be a music system available, which can be used as long as this is not loud enough to drown the exercise instructions! If there is no such system, a portable cassette player can be taken along, but make sure that it is a battery-operated one. For absolute safety, stand the player on a towel, away from the splash area, and ensure that hands are dry before adjusting the controls.

The women must have access to warm showers immediately after the exercise session and to a room in which they can have a warm drink. If there is no provision for the latter, women can be asked to bring a flask with them. The drink is necessary as blood sugar levels and blood pressure may drop following exercises in water. A separate room would allow the participants to rest and discuss posture, lifting techniques, breathing or parentcraft topics after the aquanatal session.

Equipment

Most swimming pools now have brightly coloured woggles which can be used for support, are great for relaxation and above all are fun to use!

Staffing

Adequate staffing levels are an important safety precaution. At least two professional staff and one lifeguard (preferably female) are needed at every session unless one professional has life-saving qualifications. The professionals may be a women's health physiotherapist and a midwife or, if this is not possible, two midwives may run the sessions, provided one has aquanatal qualifications. In the latter case, the exercise content should be discussed with a women's health physiotherapist beforehand. The assistant midwife will be in the water with the women to assist and correct.

Clothing

Women may wear anything comfortable, for example, maternity swimsuit, leotard or bikini with 'T'shirt over the top. It is recommended, however, that they also wear a sports bra for extra support of the breasts. The physiotherapist or midwife who is on the pool-side should wear a loose-fitting cotton 'T' shirt over a swimsuit, or possibly legging-type bottoms which will allow correct postures to be seen easily by the group. Non-slip trainer-type footwear is essential.

Antenatal

Any session should always start with a general warm-up routine, which may be carried out in or outside the pool. The warm-up serves to start to increase the load on the cardiovascular system, to mobilise the joints and to keep the body warm if the water is rather cool. This part of the routine can last up to 10 minutes.

The following input will be in the water and can include some moderate aerobic work intended to increase the heart rate and so improve cardiovascular efficiency. Care should be taken not to allow the women to exercise too strenuously as this could raise the body temperature in over-warm water and be potentially harmful for the baby (see p162). However when exercising in water of 30°C, body heat is evenly and effectively dissipated so maternal temperature is very unlikely to exceed 37° centigrade.

The aerobic part of the session can include:

- circulatory exercises
- transversus and pelvic tilting exercises
- posture
- pelvic-floor exercises
- squatting
- gentle pelvic rotation
- muscle stretching – including hip adductors
- swimming.

The above should not continue for more than half an hour, gradually slowing down with stretching, before a period of general relaxation in the pool using adequate floats. If the water is not as warm as recommended, it would be wiser to omit the relaxation period in the pool.

Postnatal

Diastasis must be excluded before performing any trunk rotations post-natally (see Ch. 8). Stretching need not include the hip adductors. All other exercises may be performed more quickly than in the antenatal period.

Points to remember when teaching aquanatal exercise

- For any trunk movements, the level of the water must reach the xiphisternum to ensure the abdominal corset is supported by the water.
- Even though the abdominal corset is protected by the hydrostatic force of the water, any rotation exercises should be performed with great care to avoid the possibility of diastasis of the recti (see Ch. 3).
- The speed at which movements are performed in water affects the difficulty of the activity – the faster the movement, the harder the work. This knowledge can be used to progress individuals postnatally.
- Care must be taken to avoid overtiring the women as they may not realise the workload they are undertaking and become fatigued. They should feel pleasantly exhilarated not exhausted.
- Exercise in water must not take place directly after a meal as cramp of the extremities is more likely when digestion is taking place. If it is not possible to arrange the session for mid-morning or afternoon, advice must be given to the women to have a light carbohydrate-rich snack about an hour before the start.
- Toe-pointing exercises should be avoided as they often lead to cramp during pregnancy.

Safeguards for the professionals

This is a list of points that should be agreed when planning aquanatal sessions (you may wish to add others):

- women to be at least 16 weeks gestation
- women to be screened correctly
- no contra-indications should be present
- a comprehensive record of appropriate personal and obstetric details to be kept
- correct pool temperature to be maintained
- check safety of pool surrounds and access to emergency telephone
- pool regulations must be observed
- ideally two professional staff and a lifeguard should be present at all times if neither professional has a lifesaving qualification
- ideal maximum number of 10–12 women
- the group to be strictly observed at all times
- no more than forty minutes of exercise to be performed
- fatigue, chill and overheating to be avoided
- women not to be allowed to over-exert themselves and produce pain
- avoid increased lumbar lordosis
- warm drink to be available afterwards.

Midwives, health visitors or physiotherapists who would like to set up aquanatal classes in their area will need to investigate local venues, contact their manager about support, funding, cover, insurance, discuss advertising methods and decide on policy, screening procedures and relevant forms. Midwives and health visitors must consult their women's health physiotherapist regarding specific exercise to be included in a session, as exercises which are normally performed on dry land need to be modified when performed in water. The leader of the sessions should be able to swim and ideally, would hold at least the Bronze Medallion in life-saving techniques.

Aquanatal sessions are beneficial during pregnancy and postnatally and encourage a healthy life style for the family where baby and family sessions are held. Above all THEY ARE FUN!

PILATES

Pilates is a mind-body technique that aims to train correct body alignment and efficient co-activation of the central core in functional activities of daily living (Stanko 2002). It is based on strength and relaxation, balancing muscle strength and flexibility. The prime postural muscles worked are the abdominals, particularly transversus, multifidus, the upper trapezii, the pelvic floor and the diaphragm, all of which are important to antenatal women and for the rehabilitation of postnatal women.

The original workout designed by Joseph Pilates consists of 34 exercises but these are not suitable for pregnancy. Modifications to the regime should be made for pregnant and postnatal women by Pilates instructors who are members of the Pilates Institute or have been trained by Body Control Pilates and who have undergone further training for pregnancy and postpartum. Women must be advised to ensure the classes they attend have been adapted for pregnancy and postpartum.

The eight principles of Pilates are:

1. concentration between mind and body
2. breathing
3. centring to create alignment and balance
4. control of movement
5. precision of each exercise
6. flowing movement
7. isolation of muscle groups
8. routine to improve muscle strength.

Pilates fits in very nicely with the concept of muscle balance, core stability and maintenance of postural alignment in all positions using the deep postural muscles. It does not encourage vigorous exercise so there is no danger of overheating; instead the movements are slow and controlled and specific.

The usual contra-indications to exercise in pregnancy and postpartum must be observed. Before resuming or taking up Pilates postnatally, the recti should be assessed to exclude any diastasis and only transversus and the pelvic floor muscles should be exercised before six weeks postpartum or longer after a caesarean delivery.

Potential benefits of Pilates during pregnancy include abdominal strength to support the uterus and help to splint the spine, improved posture and body awareness which may reduce backache and the likelihood of separated recti, improved venous return and increased stamina and energy. Pilates increases psychological well-being and self-confidence which in turn aids relaxation and sleep (see Box 12.10).

Box 12.10   Potential benefits of Pilates during pregnancy include:

- abdominal strength to support the uterus and splint the spine
- less likelihood of separated recti
- improved posture controls pelvic tilt
- reduced backache
- increased venous return
- increased stamina
- increased body awareness, aids relaxation, sleep and energy levels
- increased psychological well-being and self confidence.

Potential benefits for labour include improved abdominal strength and stamina, increased awareness of the pelvic floor to allow relaxation during childbirth and breathing techniques. Some exercises can be performed immediately postnatally which will help to realign separated rectus muscles (see Box 12.11).

Box 12.11   Potential benefits of Pilates for labour and postpartum include:

- increased awareness of pelvic floor allows relaxation to facilitate childbirth
- breathing technique helps prepare for labour
- improved abdominal strength aids childbirth
- increased stamina for labour
- realigns separated recti postnatally
- some exercises can be performed immediately postnatally.

SUMMARY OF ADVICE FOR EXERCISE TEACHERS

- Check there are no obstetric complications or pre-existing disease.
- Avoid hyperthermia, especially during the first trimester.

- Start activity slowly – warm up – build up the exercises and then cool down gradually.
- Exercise one area of the body and change to a different area for the next movement.
- Avoid positions which increase lumbar lordosis or stress on the symphysis pubis or sacroiliac joints.
- Ensure that exercises are performed slowly and accurately.
- Ensure that those women who are not accustomed to exercise do not over-exercise initially – little and often is the ideal.
- Encourage women to take time, to stretch, and get up slowly after relaxing.

SUMMARY OF ADVICE FOR WOMEN

- avoid exercising if feeling unwell
- avoid vigorous exercise in hot weather
- drink frequently whilst exercising
- avoid lying flat on the back after the fourth month of pregnancy
- listen to their bodies – if they feel dizzy or very breathless, STOP AND REST
- stop before they feel tired
- avoid holding the breath during an exercise
- exercise within the limits of individual comfort and ability
- start with a few repetitions and gradually increase
- if they feel pain – STOP
- remember that as pregnancy advances, the level of exercise will decrease.

NB. All teachers of exercise-to-music, aquanatal exercise and Pilates should be fully qualified to do so by attending an approved course and reaching the required standard of a recognised body in these fields. Women should only be directed to classes run by qualified professionals.

REFERENCES

ACOG 2002 Committee Opinion: Exercise during pregnancy and the postpartum period. Obstetrics and Gynecology 99;(1):171–173
ACPWH 1995 Guidelines for Aquanatal Classes. Association of Chartered Physiotherapists in Women's Health
Artal R, Buckenmeyer P J 1995 Exercise during pregnancy and postpartum. Contemporary Obstetrics/Gynecology 40(5):62–90
Ashton J 1992 Antenatal and postnatal classes with a difference. Journal of the Association of Chartered Physiotherapists in Obstetrics and Gynaecology 70:15–16
Brenner I K, Wolfe L A, Monga M et al 1999 Physical conditioning effects on fetal heart responses to graded maternal exercise. Medicine and Science in Sports and Exercise 31(6):792–797

Bush A 1992 Cardiopulmonary effects of pregnancy and labour. Journal of the Association of Chartered Physiotherapists in Obstetrics and Gynaecology 71:3–4

Clapp J F 3rd 2000 Exercise during pregnancy. A clinical update. Clinics in Sports Medicine Apr;(2):273–286

Clapp J F 3rd, Kim H, Burcin B, Lopez B 2000 Beginning regular exercise in early pregnancy: effect on fetoplacental growth. American Journal of Obstetrics and Gynecology 183(6):1484–1488

Dewey K G 1998 Effects of maternal caloric restriction and exercise during lactation. Journal of Nutrition 128(2 suppl): 386S–389S

Ezmerli N M 2000 Exercise in pregnancy. Primary Care Update Obstetrics and Gynaecology (1) 7(6): 260–265

Fly A D, Uhlin K L, Wallace J P 1998 Major mineral concentrations in human milk do not change after maximal exercise testing. American Journal of Clinical Nutrition 1998 68(2):345–349

Goodwin A, Astbury J, McMeeken J 2000 Body image and psychological well-being in pregnancy. A comparison of exercisers and non-exercisers. Australian and New Zealand Journal of Obstetrics and Gynaecology 40(4):442–447

Hammer R L, Perkins J, Parr R 2000 Exercise during the childbearing year. Journal of Perinatal Education 9(1):1–13

Hartman S, Bung P 1999 Physical exercise during pregnancy – physiological considerations and recommendations. Journal of Perinatal Medicine 27(3):204–215

Henriksson-Larsen K 1999 Training and sports competition during pregnancy and after childbirth. Lakartidningen 96(17):2097–2100

Jones J 2000 Exercise in pregnancy: a review of the research and a guide to advising women. Journal of the Association of Chartered Physiotherapists in Women's Health 87:9–16

Kent T, Gregor J, Deardorff L et al 1999 Edema of pregnancy: a comparison of water aerobics and static immersion. Obstetrics and Gynecology 94(5pt1):726–729

Kihlstrand M, Stennan B, Nilsson S et al 1999 Water-gymnastics reduced the intensity of back/low back pain in pregnant women. Acta Obstetrica et Gynecologica Scandinavica 78(3):180–185

Kramer M S 2002 Regular aerobic exercise during pregnancy. In the Cochrane Library, Issue 1, Oxford: Update Software

MacPhail A, Davies G A, Victory R et al 2000 Maximal exercise testing in late gestation: fetal response. Obstetrics and Gynecology 96(4):565–570

McCrory M A, Nommsen-Rivers L A, Mole P A et al 1999 Randomised trial of the short term effects of dieting plus aerobic exercise on lactation performance. American Journal of Clinical Nutrition 69(5):959–967

McMurray R G, Berry M J, Katz V 1990 The beta endorphin responses of pregnant women during aerobic exercise in the water. Medicine and Science in Sports and Exercise 22(3):298–301

O'Neill M E 1996 Maternal temperature and fetal heart rate responses to upright cycling in late pregnancy. British Journal of Sports Medicine 30(1):32–35

Polden M, Mantle J 1990 Physiotherapy in Obstetrics and Gynaecology. Butterworth Heinemann, Oxford

Revelli A, Durando A, Massobrio M 1992 Exercise and pregnancy: A review of maternal and fetal effects. Obstetrical and Gynecological Survey 47(6):355–367

Riemann M K, Kanstrup Hansen I L 2000 Effects in the foetus of exercise in pregnancy. Scandinavian Journal of Medical Sciences 10(1):12–19

Sady S P, Carpenter M W 1989 Aerobic exercise during pregnancy. Special considerations. Sports Medicine 7(6):357–375

Sampselle C M, Seng J, Yeo S et al 1999 Physical activity and postpartum well-being. Journal of Obstetrics Gynecology and Neonatal Nursing 28(1):41–49

Stanko E 2002 The role of modified Pilates in women's health physiotherapy. Journal of the Association of Chartered Physiotherapists in Women's Health 90:21–32

Wallace J P, Wiswell R A 1991 Maternal cardiovascular responses to exercise in pregnancy. In: Artal Mittlemark R, Wiswell R A, Drinkwater B (eds) Exercise in Pregnancy 2nd edn. Williams & Wilkins, Baltimore

Yeo S, Steel N M, Chang M C et al 2000 Effect of exercise on blood pressure in pregnant women with a high risk of gestational hypertensive disorders. Journal of Reproductive Medicine 45(4):93–298

Zhang J, Savitz D A 1996 Exercise during pregnancy among US women. Annals of Epidemiology 6(1):53–59

FURTHER READING

Association of Chartered Physiotherapists in Women's Health 1995 Guidelines for Aquanatal Classes. (Available from ACPWH leaflet secretary, c/o CSP, 14 Bedford Row, London WC1 4ED)

Baum G 1998 Aquarobics: the training manual. WB Saunders, London

Campion M R, Pattmann J 2002 Hydrotherapy: principles and practice 2nd edn. Butterworth Heinemann, Oxford

Evans G M 2002 Aquanatal exercise In: Campion M R, Pattman J (eds) Hydrotherapy: principles and practice 2nd edn Butterworth Heinemann, Oxford

---

VIDEOS

Pregnancy and Postnatal Exercise Video. Ashton J, Conley R, Polden M 1991 BBC Publications

Y Plan Before and After Pregnancy Video. Gaskell J, Jennings M 1991 London Central YMCA

Pilates for Pregnancy Video. Jackson L 2001 Enhance Productions, 8 RabyPark, Wetherby, LS22 6SA, Yorkshire

Suppliers of equipment and information

ITEM 171
  Leaflets 171
  Mats 172
  Models 172
  Pelvic supports 172
  Transcutaneous Electrical Nerve
    Stimulators (TENS) 172

Videos 173
Wedges 173
Wrist-splints 173
Useful Addresses 174

ITEM

NAME & ADDRESS

Anatomical Charts

Adam Rouilly Ltd, Crown Quay Lane,
Sittingbourne, Kent MElO 3JG
Tel: 01795 471378

Birthing Ball

Active Birth Centre,
25 Bickerton Road,
London N19 5JT
Tel: 020 7281 6760

Leaflets

Aquanatal Guidelines

ACPWH Leaflet Secretary,
c/o CSP, 14 Bedford Row,
London WC1R 4ED
Tel: 020 7306 6666

Fit for Pregnancy

Ralph Allen Press,
22 Milk Street

Fit for Motherhood

Bath BA1 1UT

Fit for Birth

Promoting Continence with Physiotherapy

The Mitchell Method of Simple Relaxation

Symphysis Pubis Dysfunction

Professional Affairs CSP,
14 Bedford Row,
London WC1R 4ED
Tel: 071 242 1941

Mats

Airex

CME,
7 Ascot Park Estate,
Lenton Street,
Sandiacre, Nottingham,
NG1O 5DL
Tel: 01602 390949

Nomeq,
23/24 Thornhill Road,
Redditch,
Worcestershire,
B98 9ND
Tel: 01527 64222

Models

Embryological development

Fetal doll

Pelvic floor

Pelvis

Adam Rouilly Ltd,
Crown Quay Lane,
Sittingbourne,
Kent ME10 3JG
Tel: 01795 471378

Pelvic supports

Fembrace – pelvic support

Tubigrip

Seton Products Ltd,
Turbiton House,
Oldham OL1 3H5
Tel: 0161 652 2222

Promedic pelvic support

Trochanteric Belt

Promedics Ltd,
Clarendon Road,
Blackburn,
Lancs. BB1 9TA
Tel: 01254 57700

Transcutaneous Electrical Nerve Stimulators (TENS)

Promedics Spectrum

Promedics Ltd,
Clarendon Road,
Blackburn,
Lancs. BB1 9TA
Tel: 01254 57700

Spembly Pulsar

Spembly Medical Ltd,
Newbury Road,
Andover,
Hants. SP10 4DR
Tel: 01264 65741

Videos

*The BBC Pregnancy and Postnatal
Exercise Video by ACPWH members
The Y Plan Before and After
Pregnancy Video
by YMCA*

ACPWH Leaflet Secretary,
c/o CSP,
14 Bedford Row,
London WC1R 4ED
Tel: 071 242 1941

*Pilates in Pregnancy Video by
Lindsey Jackson*

Enhance Productions,
8 Raby Park,
Wetherby LS22 6SA
Tel: 01937 586685

Wedges

Right angled

Harrison Bedding Co,
Westland Road,
Leeds LS 11
Tel: 0113 2771255

Nottingham Rehab,
Ludlow Hill Rd,
West Bridgford,
Nottingham NG2 6HD
Tel: 0115 9452345

Wrist-splints

Futura wrist-splint

Promedics Ltd,
Clarendon Road,
Blackburn,
Lancs BB1 9TA
Tel: 01254 57700

Seton Healthcare Group,
Turbiton House,
Oldham OL1 3HS
Tel: 0161 652 2222

Useful Addresses

Active Birth Centre,
25 Bickerton Road,
London N19 5JT
Tel: 020 7281 6760
www.activebirthcentre.com

Association of Chartered Physiotherapists
  in Women's Health,
c/o CSP 14, Bedford Row,
London WC1R 4ED
Tel: 020 7306 6666
www.womensphysio.com

Chartered Society of Physiotherapy,
14, Bedford Row,
London WC1R 4ED
Tel: 020 7306 6666
www.csp.org.uk

Health Visitors Association (HVA),
40 Bermondsey St,
London SE1 3UD
Tel: 020 7939 7000
www.msfcphva.org

National Childbirth Trust (NCT),
Alexandra House,
Oldham Terrace, Acton,
London W3 6NH
Tel: 0870 444 8707
www.nct-online.org/

Nursing & Midwifery Council
  (previously UKCC),
23 Portland Place,
London W1B 1PZ
Tel: 020 7333 6550
www.nmc-uk.org/cms

Royal College of Midwives (RCM),
15 Mansfield Street,
London W1G 9NH
Tel: 020 7291 9220/1
www.rcm.org.uk

Index

Note:
Page numbers in **bold,** refer to major discussions.
Page numbers in *italics,* refer to figures.

Abdominal exercises, 45–47
  antenatal, 45–47
    teaching, *123,* 122–127, *123, 124,*
      125, 126
  pelvic tilting (rocking), 22, 26, 46–47, *47*
  post-caesarean, 111
  postpartum, 104–106, *106,* 111
    teaching, *130,* 130–134, *130, 132, 133*
  transversus, 45–46, *46, 104,* 104–105
Abdominal muscles, 4–11
  combined functions, 11
  external oblique, 4, *7, 7–8, 10,* 11
  internal oblique, 4, 5–6, *6, 10,* 11
  multifidus, 9–10
  nerve supply, 11
  pyramidalis, 9
  rectus abdominis, 8, *9–10*
  rectus sheath, 8, 10, *10*
  transversus abdominis, 4–5, *5, 9*
Abdominal wall, 4–11
  fascia, 4, 8, 10
  linea alba, 4, *5–7, 9*
  muscles, 4–11
Addresses for information, 174
Aerobic exercises, 158–160
  antenatal, 42, 158–159
  clothing, 160
  facilities and equipment, 159–160
  postpartum, 159
Antenatal class planning *see* Programme
  planning for physical skills
Antenatal exercises and advice, **41–56**
  abdominal exercises, 45–47
  aerobic exercises, 158–159
  aquanatal exercises, 160–166
  backcare, 47–54, 145
  exercises to avoid, *55,* 55–56
  foot and leg exercises, *42,* 42–43
  household activities, 53–54, *53–54*

  lifting, 52, *52–53*
  lying, 50, *50–51*
  pelvic floor exercises, 44–45, 46
  pelvic tilting, 22, 26, 44–47, *46–47, 47*
  pilates, 166–167
  shoulder, arm and chest exercises,
    137–138
  sitting postures, 48, *48*
  standing, 49, *49*
  stretching exercises, 54
  teaching, **120–127**
  transversus exercises, 45–46, *46*
  see also Exercise in pregnancy; *individual*
    exercises
Antenatal team, 143–144
Aponeurosis, 4, *6, 7, 8, 9*
Aquanatal exercise, 160–166
  antenatal, 42, 164
  benefits, 160–161
  clothing, 164
  contraindications, 161–162
  equipment, 163
  facilities, 162–163
  postnatal, 164
  potential dangers in pregnancy, 163
  safeguards for professionals, 165–166
  teaching points, 165
Aromatherapy, 66
Assisted delivery
  exercises after, **109**

Backache, 95
Backcare, antenatal advice, 47–54, 145
  postnatal advice, 112–114
Back pain, *see* Low back pain
Birthing cushion, 74
Birthing partner, 77–78, 146–147
Birthing positions *see* Labour, positions

Bowel problems, 97
Breastfeeding
 positions for, 109, *112*
Breathing
 awareness, 145–146
 pant-pant-blow, 74
 relaxation, 63–64, 71, 145–146
 second stage, 77
 sighing out slowly (SOS), 72, 79
 in threes, 74
 see also Respiration; Respiratory system
Breathlessness (dyspnoea), 15–16
Bulbospongiosus, 11, *12*

Caesarean section/delivery, 109–111
 abdominal exercises, 111
 antenatal/postnatal class planning, 147
 foot and leg exercises, 110
 pelvic floor exercises, 111
 post-operative pain relief, 88–89
 postpartum exercises and advice,
  109–111, *110*, *111*
 wound haematoma, 94
Cardiovascular system, 16–17
 changes in postpartum, 92
 changes in pregnancy, 16–17
Carpal tunnel syndrome, 17, 21
Circulatory exercises *see* Diaphragmatic
  breathing; Foot and leg exercises
Coccydynia, 95–96
Coccygeus, 12, *13*
Cold therapy, bruised and oedematous
  perineum, 93–94
Collagen elasticity in pregnancy, 17
Constipation, 97
Contractions *see* Labour, contractions
Coping strategies, in labour, **70–77**
 teaching, 69, 78–80
Core trunk stability exercises, 106–109
 postpartum, 106–109, *107*, *107*, *109*
 teaching, *134*, 134–137, *135*, *136*
Couples, programme planning for physical
  skills, 146–147
Cramp, 20, 78
Cystocoele, 37

Daily activities, 112, *114*
Deep venous thrombosis, 101
Delivery positions *see* Labour, positions
Diaphragm, positional variations, 16
Diaphragmatic breathing, 102
Diastasis recti, 18, 31–34, 94–95
 advice for women, 34
 incidence, 31–32, 92
 labour positions, 76
 rectus check, 33
 treatment, 33

Diastasis symphysis pubis *see* Symphysis
  pubis dysfunction (SPD)
Dyspareunia, 97
Dyspnoea, 15–16

Encephalins, 83
Endorphins, 83, 85
Epidural anaesthesia, 77, 101
 foot and leg exercises after, 101
 low back pain, 26, 95
Episiotomy, 77, 97
Ethnic minorities, 148
Exercise in pregnancy, alternative
  approaches, **153–170**
 benefits, 153–155
 cardiovascular, 156
 contraindications, 157
 physiology, 154
 postulated dangers, 155–156
 risk activities, 156–157
 risk groups, 157–158
 safety precautions, 157–158
 summary of advice, 167–168
  teachers, 167–168
  women, 168
 see also Antenatal exercises and advice
Exercises to avoid, 55–56, 115
 antenatal, 55–56
 postpartum, 115
Exercise teaching *see* Teaching (of) exercises
External anal sphincter, 11, *12*
External oblique muscle, 4, *7*, *7–8*, *10*, 11

Faecal incontinence, 37, 97
 treatment, 37
Fascia
 pelvic, 13, 92
 thoracolumbar, 10
Fatigue, 16, 22, 97–98
Fight-flight response, 57–59, *59*
Foot and leg exercises, 42–43, 101–102,
  102, 110
 antenatal, *42*, 42–43
  teaching, *120*, 120–121
 post-caesarean, 110
 postpartum, 101–102, *102*, 110
  teaching, 127–128, *128*
Footwear advice, 43
Forceps deliveries, 74, 109
 faecal incontinence risk, 37

Genital prolapse *see* Prolapse

Haematoma, 94
Haemorrhoids, 17, 94

Historical perspectives, ix–xi
  physical preparation for childbirth,
    ix–xi
Hormonal effect (pregnancy), 15
  bladder and urethra, 19
  cardiovascular system, 16–17
  collagen, 17
  diastasis recti, 31–32
  lactation, 91
  linea alba, 4, 31, 92
  low back pain, 25–26
  musculoskeletal system, 17–19, 92,
    144, 155
  pelvic floor, 92
  respiratory system, 15
  stress, 60
  symphysis pubis dysfunction, 30, 95
Household activities advice, 53–54, *53, 54*
Hyperventilation, 70–71
  maternal, 15–16
  prevention in labour, 69, 70–71, 74
Hypnosis, 66
Hypotension, supine, 17

Iliococcygeus, 12, *13*
Ischiocavernosus, 11, *13*
Imagery and suggestion, 66–67
Incontinence, 35–37
  see also Faecal incontinence; Urinary
    incontinence
Internal oblique muscle, 4, 5–6, *6, 10,* 11
  actions, 6
Ischiococcygeus, 12, *13*

Joints, laxity, 17–18

Kyphosis, 18

Labour, **69–81**
  breathing, 70–71, 72, 74, 79
  contractions, 79–80
  coping strategies, **70–77**
  crowning, 77, 80
  first stage, 78–79
  hyperventilation prevention, 69,
    70–71, 74
  pain management *see* Pain management
  positions, 73–77, *74, 75, 76*
    diastasis symphysis pubis, 76
    end of first stage, 73–74, *74*
    first stage, 71–72, *73*
    second stage, 74–77, *75, 76*
    women with special needs, 76
  problems, 69–70
  rehearsal, 78–81

  relaxation during, 64, 72
  role of partner, 77–78
  second stage
    teaching coping strategies, 69, **78–80**
    see also Relaxation, teaching
  TENS *see* Transcutaneous electrical nerve
    stimulation (TENS)
Lactation, 91
Leg exercises *see* Foot and leg exercises
Leg-tightening, 43, *43*, 102
Levator ani, 12, *13*
Lifting advice, 52, *52–53*, 113
Ligaments, pelvic
Linea alba, 4, *5, 6, 7, 9,* 10, 17, 31
Low back pain (LBP), 18, 22, 25–27, 95
  acute, management, 22
  advice for women, 27
  epidural anaesthesia and, 26
  hormonal factors, 25–26
  postnatal, 26–27
  predisposing factors, 25–26
  treatment, 26–27
Lumbar lordosis, *19*, 155
Lying posture, 43, 50, *50, 51*

Massage, 66, 78, 147
Median nerve compression, 21
Muscle imbalance, 26, 30, 129
Multifidus, 9–10
Musculoskeletal problems, in pregnancy
    and postpartum, **25–40**
  diastasis recti, 31–34
  faecal incontinence, 37
  low back pain, 25–27
  pelvic floor dysfunction, 35–38
  posterior pelvic pain, 27–28
  pregnancy-associated osteoporosis,
    34–35
  prolapse, 25, 37–38
  symphysis pubis dysfunction, 20–21,
    28–31, 95
  urinary incontinence, 35–37
  see also individual conditions
Musculoskeletal system, 17–20, 92
  changes in postpartum, 92
  changes in pregnancy, 17–20
  hormonal effects, 17–19, 92, 144, 155

Nerve supply
  abdominal muscles, 11
  pelvic floor, 13

Oblique muscle (abdominal)
  external, 4, *7, 7–8, 10,* 11
  internal *see* Internal oblique muscle
Oestrogen, 15, 17

Osteoporosis, pregnancy-associated *see*
  Pregnancy-associated osteoporosis
  (PAO)

Pain management, 93–94, 95–96, 97
  cold therapy, 93–94
  pulsed electromagnetic energy *see* Pulsed
    electromagnetic energy (PEME)
  therapeutic ultrasound, 94, 97
Pelvic floor, 11–14
  anatomy, 11–14, *12, 13*
  dysfunction, 35–38, 92
    faecal incontinence, 37
    prolapse, 37–38
    urinary incontinence, 35–37
  fascia, 13, 92
  levator ani, 12, *13*
  muscles, combined functions, 13–14
  nerve supply, 13
    damage and faecal incontinence, 37
  superficial perineal muscles, 11, *12*
Pelvic floor exercises, 44–45, 46, 102–104
  antenatal, 44–45, 46
    teaching, 121–122
  post-caesarean, 111
  postpartum, 102–104
    teaching, *128*, 128–130
  prolapse treatment, 37–38
  transversus and, 46
  urinary incontinence reduction, 35–37
    stress incontinence, 36
Pelvic support, belt, girdle, 22, 27, 28, 30
Pelvic ligaments, anterior/posterior view, *2, 3*
Pelvic stability, 2
  core stability exercises, 106–109, *107,
    107, 109*
  teaching, *134*, 134–137, *135, 136*
Pelvic tilting (rocking) exercises, 46–47
  antenatal, 22, 26, 46–47, *47*
    teaching, 124–127, *125, 126*
  method, 46–47, *47*
  postpartum, 105, *106*
Pelvis, 1
  anatomical relations, 3–4
  anatomy, *1–14*
  closing mechanisms, 2
  diameter changes
  joints, 1, 2
    hormonal pliability, 2
    stability, 2
Perineal body, 11, *12*
Perineum, 74–75, 93–94
  bruised and oedematous postpartum,
    93–94
    cold therapy application, 93
    pulsed electromagnetic energy
      application, 94

  therapeutic ultrasound application, 94
Physical problems, postpartum, **93–100**
  backache, 95
  bowel problems, 97
  bruised and oedematous perineum, 93–94
  coccydynia, 95–96
  diastasis recti, 94–95
    see also Diastasis recti
  dyspareunia, 97
  fatigue, 97–98
  haematoma, 94
  haemorrhoids, 94
  symphysis pubis dysfunction, 95
    see also Symphysis pubis dysfunction
      (SPD)
  urinary problems, 96–97
  see also Musculoskeletal problems, in
    pregnancy and postpartum
Physical problems in pregnancy, **20–23**
  breathlessness (dyspnoea), 16
  carpal tunnel syndrome, 21
  cramp, 20, 78
  hyperventilation, 15–16
  low back pain *see* Low back pain (LBP)
  rib-flaring, 16, 18, 21
  rib-pain (stitch), 21
  stress incontinence, 21–22
  symphysis pubis dysfunction, 20–21,
    28–31, 95
    see also Symphysis pubis dysfunction
      (SPD)
  tiredness (fatigue), 16, 22, 97–98
  varicose veins, 17, 20
  see also Musculoskeletal problems, in
    pregnancy and postpartum
Physiological changes in postpartum, **91–92**
  cardiovascular system, 92
  musculoskeletal system, 92
Physiological changes in pregnancy, **15–20**
  cardiovascular system, 16–17
  musculoskeletal system, 17–20
  respiratory system, 15–16
  see also individual systems and changes
Pilates, 166–167
  potential benefits, 167
Posterior pelvic pain (PPP), 27–28
  advice for women, 28
  treatment, 28
Postnatal *see Entries beginning* postpartum
Postpartum class planning *see* Programme
  planning for physical skills
Postpartum exercises and advice, **101–116**
  abdominal exercises, *104*, 104–106, *106*
    post-caesarean, 111
  aerobic exercises, 159
  aquanatal exercises, 160–166
  assisted delivery, 109
  avoidance exercises, 115

backcare, 112–114
caesarean delivery, 109–111, *111*
classes, 115–116
core trunk stability exercises, 106–109,
   107, 109
foot and leg exercises, 101–102, *102*
   post-caesarean, 110
household activities, 114
lifting, 112–114
pelvic floor exercises, 102–104
   post-caesarean, 111
pelvic tilting exercises, 105, *106*
pilates, 166–167
rectus check, 105–106
teaching, **127–137**, 146
transversus exercises, *104,* 104–105
see also Exercise in pregnancy; *individual*
   exercises
Postpartum period, problems in *see*
   Musculoskeletal problems; Physical
   problems, postpartum
Posture/positions, 47–54
getting-up, *51*
household activities, 53–54, *51–53, 54*
labour *see* Labour, positions
lifting, *52, 53*
lying, 43, 50, *50–51*
normal, *19*
in pregnancy, 18, *19*
relaxed, 61, *62*
sitting, 43, 48, *48*
standing, 49, *49*
stress, *58,* 58–59
see also Postpartum exercises and advice,
   backcare
Pregnancy, problems in *see* Musculoskeletal
   problems; Physical problems in
   pregnancy
Pregnancy-associated osteoporosis (PAO),
   34–35
causes, 35
characteristics, 34–35
Problems in postpartum *see*
   Musculoskeletal problems; Physical
   problems, postpartum
Problems in pregnancy *see* Musculoskeletal
   problems; Physical problems in
   pregnancy
Progesterone, 15, 16
Programme planning for physical skills,
   143–152
antenatal team composition, 143–144
attendance, 144–145
caesarean delivery, 147
content of antenatal and postpartum
   classes, 144–151
couples, 146–147
early pregnancy, 144–145

ethnic minorities, 148
health and safety precautions, 144
individuals, 149
postpartum classes, 149–150
   community, 150
   reunion, 150
refreshers, 149
special needs women, 149
teenager's clubs, 148
TENS, 147–148
ward classes, 149
women only, 145–146
see also Teaching exercises
Prolactin, 91
Prolapse (genital), 25, 37–38
prevention, 44
treatment, 37–38
Psychoprophylaxis, 70, ix
See also Respiration
Pubococcygeus, 12, *13*
Puborectalis, 12, *13*
Puerperium *see Entries beginning* postpartum
Pulsed electromagnetic energy (PEME), 94
bruised and oedematous perineum, 94
coccydynia, 95–96
haematoma and haemorrhoids, 94
Pulsed shortwave *see* Pulsed
   electromagnetic energy (PEME)
Pyramidalis, 9
implication in diastasis recti, 31–32

Rectocoele, 37
Rectus abdominis, 8, *9, 10,* 18
actions, 8
diastasis recti *see* Diastasis recti
Rectus check, 33, 105–106
Rectus sheath, 8, *10,* 17
Relaxation, **60–67**
aromatherapy, 66
hypnosis, 66
imagery and suggestion, 66–67
during labour, 64, 72
massage, 66
passive/active, 63, 64, 65
physiological, 61–65
   technique, 61–63
position/posture of ease, *50,* 61, *62*
   first stage of labour, 71–72, *73*
reciprocal, 61
teaching, 64–65
   see also Labour, teaching coping
     strategies
touch, 65–66
transcendental meditation (TSM), 67
yoga, 67
Relaxin, 15, 17, 92, 155
increase linked to low back pain, 25–26

Relaxin (*continued*)
musculoskeletal changes, 17–18
posterior pelvic pain association, 27
sites of action, 17
symphysis pubis dysfunction, 30
Respiration
control, 70
diaphragmatic, 102
hyperventilation prevention, 70–71, 72
in labour, 70–71
relaxation, 63–64, 71, 145–146
Respiratory system, 15–16
changes in pregnancy, 15–16, 155
in exercise, 70
in labour, 70–71
stress and tension effect, 58–59
Rib-flaring, 16, 18, 21
Rib-pain (stitch), 21

Sacroiliac joint, 1, 2
Sciatica, 27
Shoulder, arm and chest exercises,
antenatal, 137–138
Sighing out slowly breathing (SOS), 72, 79
Sitting posture, 43, 48, *48*
Slow-twitch type I muscle fibres, 45, 103
SOS breathing, 72, 79
Special needs women, 76, 149
antenatal programme planning, 149
labour positions, 76
Spine, 2, 11, 18
backcare
antenatal, 47–54, 145
postpartum, 112–114
kyphosis, 18
pain in *see* Low back pain (LBP)
stability, 2, 11
core stability exercises, 106–109, *107, 109*
teaching, *134,* 134–137, *135, 136*
Standing posture, 49, *49*
Stress, **57–60**
coping with, 60
see also Relaxation
fetus/newborn, effect on, 60
'fight or flight,' 57–59, *59,* 64
in labour, 69–70
physiological changes, 58–59
in pregnancy, 59–60
tension position/posture, 58, *58*
see also Relaxation
Stress incontinence, 21–22, 36, 96
Stretching exercises, antenatal, 54
teaching, 138–142, *139, 140, 141*
warning, 141–142
Superficial perineal muscles, 11, *12*
Supine hypotension, 17
Suppliers of equipment and information,
171–174

leaflets, 171
mats, 172
models, 172
pelvic supports, 172
Transcutaneous Electric Nerve
Stimulators (TENS), 172–173
useful addresses
videos, 173
wedges, 173
wrist-splints, 173
Symphysis pubis, 1, *2, 13*
Symphysis pubis dysfunction (SPD), 20–21,
28–31, 95
advice for women, 31
characteristics/symptoms, 29
epidural anaesthesia, 30
guidelines, 31
incidence, 29
labour implications, 30
labour position, 76
treatment, 30–31
after delivery, 30–31
during labour/delivery, 30
during pregnancy, 30

Teaching (of) exercises, **117–142**
arranging the group, 118–120
useful considerations, 119
caution and advice, 117–118, 141–142,
167–168
coping strategies in labour, 69, 78–80
equipment and facilities, 118
evaluation, 137
instructions *see* individual exercises
rehearsal of labour, 78–81
relaxation, 64–65
teacher comprehension, 117–118, 120
using music, 120, 159–160, 163
see also Programme planning for physical
skills
Teenagers, 148–149
Tension *see* Stress
Therapeutic ultrasound, 94, 97
Thoracolumbar fascia, 10
Tiredness *see* Fatigue
Touch, 65–66
Transcendental meditation (TSM), 67
Transcutaneous electrical nerve stimulation
(TENS), **83–90**
advantages in labour, 84–85
antenatal/postnatal class planning,
147–148
electrodes, 85–87
hire package, 87, *88*
post-caesarean delivery, applications,
88–89
selection criteria for unit, 87–88
Transversus abdominis, 4–5, *5, 9, 10, 11*

Transversus exercises, 33, 45–46, 104–105
    antenatal, 45–46, *46*
        teaching, *123*, 123–124, *124*
    postpartum, *104*, 104–105
Trochanteric belt, 20, 30

Ultrasound, therapeutic, 94, 97
Urinary frequency, 4
Urinary incontinence, 19, 35–37, 92, 96–97
    causes/pathophysiology, 35–37
    frequency, 36
    prevention, 44
    stress, 21–22, 36, 96
    treatment/prevention, 36–37
    urgency and urge, 36
Uterus, 3–4
    muscle contractions *see* Labour,
        contractions
    nerve roots, 85

positional variations, 3–4, 16, 18
prolapse, 37
    see also Prolapse (genital)

Valsalva manoeuvre, 77
Varicose veins, 17, 20

Women's health physiotherapist, 143
    antenatal exercise/advice introduction, 41
    referrals, 31, 37–38, 97
        low back pain, 26, 27
        posterior pelvic pain, 27–28
    ultrasound or pulsed electromagnetic
        energy (PEME) administration, 94
Wrist-splints, 21

Yoga, 67